MW01119492

SEXUAL IDENTITIES AND SEXUALITY IN SOCIAL WORK

Contemporary Social Work Studies

Series Editor:
Robin Lovelock, University of Southampton, UK

Series Advisory Board:
Lena Dominelli, University of Durham, UK
Jan Fook, University of Southampton, UK
Peter Ford, University of Southampton, UK
Lorraine Gutiérrez University of Michigan, USA
Lucy Jordan, University of Southampton, UK
Walter Lorenz, Free University of Bozen-Bolzano, Italy
Patrick O'Leary, University of Southampton, UK
Joan Orme, University of Glasgow, UK
Jackie Powell, University of Southampton, UK
Gillian Ruch, University of Southampton, UK
Sue White, University of Birmingham, UK

Contemporary Social Work Studies is a series disseminating high quality new research and scholarship in the discipline and profession of social work. The series promotes critical engagement with contemporary issues relevant across the social work community and captures the diversity of interests currently evident at national, international and local levels.

CSWS is located in the School of Social Sciences (Social Work Studies Division) at the University of Southampton, UK and is a development from the successful series of books published by Ashgate in association with CEDR (the Centre for Evaluative and Developmental Research) from 1991.

Other titles in this series:

Professional Discretion in Welfare Services
Beyond Street-Level Bureaucracy
Tony Evans
ISBN 978–0–7546–7491–7

Indigenous Social Work around the World
Towards Culturally Relevant Education and Practice
Edited by Mel Gray, John Coates and Michael Yellow Bird
ISBN 978–1–4094–0794–2

For information about other titles in this series, visit www.ashgate.com

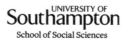

UNIVERSITY OF
Southampton
School of Social Sciences

Sexual Identities and Sexuality in Social Work

Research and Reflections from Women in the Field

Edited by

PRISCILLA DUNK-WEST
Coventry University, UK

TRISH HAFFORD-LETCHFIELD
Middlesex University, UK

ASHGATE

Published by
Ashgate Publishing Limited
Wey Court East
Union Road
Farnham
Surrey, GU9 7PT
England

Ashgate Publishing Company
Suite 420
101 Cherry Street
Burlington
VT 05401–4405
USA

www.ashgate.com

British Library Cataloguing in Publication Data
Sexual identities and sexuality in social work : research and reflections from women
    in the field. – (Contemporary social work studies)
    1. Social service and sex. 2. Social work with sexual minorities.
    3. Women social workers. 4. Feminist theory.
    I. Series. II. Dunk-West, Priscilla.
    III. Hafford-Letchfield, Trish.
    361.3'2–dc22

Library of Congress Cataloging-in-Publication Data
Sexual identities and sexuality in social work : research and reflections from women
    in the field / [edited] by Priscilla Dunk-West and Trish Hafford-Letchfield.
        p. cm. – (Contemporary social work studies)
    Includes bibliographical references and index.
    ISBN 978–0–7546–7882–3 (hbk. : alk. paper) – ISBN 978–0–7546–9745–9
    1. Social service – Research. 2. Social service – Practice. 3. Sexism. 4. Sex.
    5. Sexual orientation. I. Dunk-West, Priscilla. II. Hafford-Letchfield, Trish.
    HV11.S4754 2011
    361.3082–dc22   2010046227

ISBN 9780754678823 (hbk)
ISBN 9780754697459 (ebk)

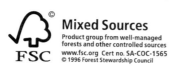

Printed and bound in Great Britain by
MPG Books Group, UK

Contents

Notes on Contributors   *vii*
Preface, Jan Fook   *xi*
Acknowledgements   *xiii*

Introduction: Sexualities and Sexual Identities in Social Work   1
Priscilla Dunk-West and Trish Hafford-Letchfield

1   Sexuality and Women in Care Organizations: Negotiating
Boundaries within a Gendered Cultural Script   11
Trish Hafford-Letchfield

2   'A Chance to Cut is a Chance to Cure': Self-harm and
Self-protection – A Gay Perspective   31
Sarah Carr

3   Researching Sexuality and Ageing   45
Rhiannon Jones

4   Reflecting on Sexual Health and Young Women's Sexuality:
Business or Pleasure?   61
Michelle Brown and Priscilla Dunk-West

5   Growing up with a Lesbian or Gay Parent: Young People's
Perspectives   71
Anna Fairtlough

6   Have you Heard? … Reflections on the Kerr/Haslam Inquiry   89
Jeanette Copperman

7   The Assessment of Lesbian and Gay Prospective Foster Carers:
Twenty Years of Practice and What has Changed?   105
Helen Cosis Brown

8   What is Personal? Reflecting on Heterosexuality   121
Joy Trotter

9   Sexuality before Ability? The Assessment of Lesbians as
     Adopters   141
     Christine Cocker

10   Identity, Emotion Work and Reflective Practice: Dealing with
     Sexuality, Race and Religion in the Classroom   163
     Cathy Aymer and Rachana Patni

11   Everyday Sexuality and Identity: De-differentiating the Sexual
     Self in Social Work   177
     Priscilla Dunk-West

Index   *193*

Notes on Contributors

Cathy Aymer is a senior lecturer in social work at Brunel University. Her background is in work with children and families. She has written extensively about anti-discriminatory practice in welfare. Her PhD research was concerned with the experiences of black professionals in white organizations. She continuously struggles with the question: how can I improve my practice as an educator?

Michelle Brown has studied human services, gender studies and family mediation. She began working with young people in 2001 providing counselling and group work services in South Australia. This was followed by a specialist role in sexual health providing young people with sexual health education, information and advice with a predominant role in health promotion. Working specifically with young women has brought her many challenges and experiences and she has continued on to various roles including specialist sexual and relationships education work and national health programmes in the United Kingdom. She is committed to providing services and working with young people and is now working as a Youth Engagement Coordinator providing opportunities to young people.

Sarah Carr is a Senior Research Analyst at the Social Care Institute for Excellence (SCIE), currently leading on the organization's personalization work and advising on the policy at a national level. She has also worked for the National Institute for Social Work, Oxleas NHS Trust and at the Sainsbury Centre for Mental Health in research and information roles. In addition to her post at SCIE, Sarah is currently an Honorary Fellow at the Faculty of Health at Staffordshire University, an Executive Committee member of the Social Perspectives Network (SPN) and a Board Member of the National Development Team for Inclusion (NDTi). She is a long-term user of mental health services and has written on her own experiences as well as general mental health practice and policy, LGB welfare and equality issues, service user empowerment and participation.

Christine Cocker is a principal lecturer in social work at Middlesex University. She is currently an independent member of a local authority adoption panel. Christine underwent her social work training in New Zealand in the 1980s. She moved to England in 1988 and worked as a social worker and a social work manager in the children and families department of an inner London borough for 13 years, before joining a voluntary sector consultation service. Christine began working at Middlesex University in 2003. Her research and publications are in the area of social work with looked after children, and lesbian and gay fostering and adoption. Her most recent book is: Cocker, C. and Allain, L. (2008) *Social Work* *with Looked After Children*, Exeter: Learning Matters. Christine published two more books in 2010: Cocker, C. and Allain, L. (2010) *Advanced Social Work with Children and Families*, Exeter: Learning Matters; and Brown, H.C. and Cocker, C. (2010) *Sexuality and Social Work: Theory and Practice*, London, Sage.

Jeanette Copperman is a senior lecturer in social work at City University, London. She currently teaches, researches and writes on interprofessional practice and on mental health issues. She began work in Botswana as a community development worker and then practised as an advice and community worker in the voluntary sector in the UK. She became a policy advisor on women's issues and then on user involvement in the health service. She has a background in mental health policy and practice and her research interests include gender, equalities in mental health, organizational change and user involvement. Her recent publications include Hammick, M., Freeth, D., Copperman, J., and Goodsman, D. (2009) *Being Interprofessional* Cambridge, Polity Press.

Helen Cosis Brown is a principal lecturer in social work at Middlesex University. She also works as an independent foster carer reviewing officer, and chairs a local authority fostering panel. She worked as a social worker and a social work manager in inner London before moving into social work education. Her publications have been about social work with lesbians and gay men as well as fostering and adoption and include Brown H.C. (1998) *Sexuality and Social Work: Working with Lesbians and Gay Men*, Basingstoke: Macmillan.

Priscilla Dunk-West is a senior lecturer in the Faculty of Health and Life Studies at Coventry University. She has been involved in sexuality research, scholarship and queer activism since her undergraduate days some twenty years ago. In her social work practice career, Priscilla worked in child protection before specializing in the area of sexual health counselling which saw her work with individuals and couples experiencing sexual problems. Her PhD in sociology focused on theorizing identity as it relates to the sexual self. Broadly speaking, her research is concerned with the sociology of everyday identities and selfhood: how these relate to the social work role is an enduring area of interest.

Anna Fairtlough is a lecturer in social work at Goldsmiths, University of London. She has many years experience as a social worker and social work educator. Her research and teaching interests lie in the fields of parenting, equalities and professional development. She is a lesbian parent herself and has been actively involved in different groups for lesbian and gay parents and their children.

Jan Fook is Professor of Professional Practice Research and Director, Interprofessional Institute, South West London Academic Network (Royal Holloway, University of London, St Georges, University of London, and Kingston University).

Trish Hafford-Letchfield is a senior lecturer at Middlesex University and has worked in higher education for a number of years, teaching on social work, social care and learning and teaching courses. Trish is a qualified nurse, social worker and teacher and has had a long career in statutory social work with the last 10 years as a manager in Adult Services. Trish has published a number of texts in the area of organizational and management development. Her current research interests are in the area of sexuality, widening participation and the lifelong learning of older people. Trish is on the National Executive of Education and Ageing and is very active in her role as Chair of her local Age Concern. In her spare time, she plays the violin in an amateur orchestra.

Rhiannon Jones is senior lecturer at Manchester Metropolitan University teaching on both undergraduate and postgraduate social work programmes. Her current teaching areas are research methods and social work with older people. Prior to this Rhiannon worked as a practitioner for over 15 years in statutory social work with adults, particularly older adults with mental health issues. Rhiannon has a strong commitment to developing critical and empowering perspectives in relation to a range of issues affecting older people. She is currently undertaking her doctoral study with Sociological Department of the University of Sheffield in her principal research area of sexuality and ageing. Rhiannon's presentations at national and international conferences have focused on issues of sexuality in relation to counselling, social work, ageing and in particular the methodological issues raised by researching sexuality in later life. In 2007 she co-authored (with Julie Bywater) *Sexuality and Social Work*, which was published by Learning Matters.

Rachana Patni is a lecturer at Brunel University, where she currently contributes to social work modules that have an applied theoretical emphasis. In this capacity she has struggled (and struggles) with pedagogical and professional socialization issues for social work students' value commitments with regard to sexuality.

Joy Trotter is reader in social work at the University of Teesside. She began her social work career in field work in 1976 and has worked at the University of Teesside since 1987 (where she was awarded a PhD in Social Work in 2003). Joy's publications include three books and over twenty articles and chapters about child sexual abuse, domestic violence, qualitative research methods, social work education and sexuality issues. In the past she has been an active member of JUCSWEC Research Sub-Committee, an editorial board member of *Social Work Education*, chair of ATSWE and co-ordinator of the National Sexuality Symposium, and is currently on the editorial board of the *British Journal of Social Work*. Most recently she has edited a Special Issue of *Social Work Education* (with Christine Knott and Sheila Kershaw) and published articles in *Research, Policy and Planning, Ethics and Social Welfare* and the *Journal of LGBT Youth*.

Preface

Jan Fook

Notions of sexuality and sexual identity are clearly aligned with key thinking and practice in social work. Priscilla Dunk-West and Trish Hafford-Letchfield make this argument convincingly in this book. In short, we need to be informed of current understandings of sexuality and sexual identity in order to practice social work effectively. The nature of intimacy and our emotional lives, how we frame gender, the identities we construct for ourselves and others, are all integral to the fundamental concerns of social work in mainstream areas such as child and family work, ageing and mental health.

It is particularly pertinent to visit and revisit the issue of identity in a constantly changing environment. The book tackles this topic pointedly, and in a refreshing and also multi-perspectival way. The combination of review and argument, empirical research and personal reflection makes a welcome contribution to the way we approach an understanding of many of the major phenomena in social work. In fact, it supports the idea that human experiences are neither solely personal nor social in nature, but must be appreciated from a number of viewpoints and using a number of different methods. This is certainly an approach for our times.

I am pleased to see the inclusion of reflective practice and reflexivity in the volume, as I do see these concepts as crucial to new and developing understandings of how we practice in a professional manner in an increasingly complex global environment. The authors use these concepts in a refreshing and sophisticated way which provides an excellent model for students and future social workers.

In addition, there is very clear inclusion of a number of new and innovative research methodologies, such as the use of life stories. Other innovative inclusions are the organizational, management and leadership perspectives, along with a focus on a change agenda. Overall then, what is provided is a definitive example of the treatment of a key topic (sexuality and sexual identity) in a multi-perspectival way, using a range of methods. It constitutes a wonderful model of how topics should be approached in contemporary social work.

Acknowledgements

We would like to thank all of the wonderful women whose chapters are contained herein: your perspectives make this collection unique and powerful. Thank you to the staff at Ashgate for their guidance and support, in particular, Claire Jarvis.

To my wonderful family of choice: Brad, Blake and Paxton.

Priscilla Dunk-West

This book is dedicated to my mum Sylvie, my daughter Katie, my sister Anne and my aunty Doreen; four exceptional women.

Trish Hafford-Letchfield

Introduction
Sexualities and Sexual Identities in Social Work

Priscilla Dunk-West and Trish Hafford-Letchfield

This book examines the relationship between social work and sexuality. It does this by showcasing a range of issues pertinent to social work which have been analysed by looking through the lens of sexuality. In this way, social work's relationship with sexuality is unravelled in *Sexual Identities and Sexuality in Social Work*. In this introduction we discuss the rationale for bringing together the different research-based and reflective contributions and we conclude by providing short synopses of each chapter.

The varied contributions to this book cut across a number of themes that can be grouped in various ways: for example, in relation to sexuality and sexual identity; family care and relationships; difference and diversity; identity and power and abuse and harm. Although we contend that sexuality is not a specialist topic or area of practice which cuts across all areas of social work, to relegate it to any one single field of practice would be very misleading. In bringing together this edited collection, we have also been mindful of the central placement of empirical and theoretical work within the social work literature. Notwithstanding the contribution such works make to our understanding of sexuality, you will find that we have interspersed theoretical and research-based chapters with more reflective pieces. This approach serves to enrich and diversify the approach to understanding and thinking about sexuality in the field. Placing research alongside critical reflection allows a unique perspective on sexuality and sexual identity to emerge, because it enables to reader to engage with different forms of knowledge in a more coherent way. Our approach echoes some of the commentary within social work about the nature of knowledge and the different tensions that exist within the discipline between practice-based wisdom and formal, theoretical knowledge (Eraut 1994). Pressure in pedagogy to orient students towards 'evidence-based practice' or 'research based practice' with less emphasis on 'practice wisdom' (Lewis 2003) is one example of the way in which the rise of professionalism has pushed increasingly risk averse frameworks to dominate. Similarly, research is bounded by rules, methods and clear processes whereas reflection is somewhat tenuous and meandering. This tension between research and reflection is made deliberately manifest in the underpinning structure of this book because we believe that the complexities inherent in sexuality and social work may emerge from marrying together these two ways of seeing.

Before introducing you to the content through a chapter-by-chapter synopsis, we first turn to a more general discussion about sexuality within the landscape of contemporary social work practice. What do we mean when we speak of sexuality and a sexual identity? Notwithstanding the subjective nature of definitions, which can be seen through the subtle differences in the ways the chapters in this edited work deal with these concepts, we are able to speak generally about these interrelated terms. Sexuality is an umbrella term that relates to the private dimension in which people live out their sexual, intimate and/or emotional desires. Sexual identity, on the other hand, suggests a stance in orientation: it provokes categorical discernment. Thus, sexual identity is akin to defining the nature of one's attractions and desires and terms that pronounce this include lesbian, gay, bisexual, queer, heterosexual and questioning. Since social work's core purpose is to work with individuals, communities and groups, it is not surprising that sexuality and sexual identity may be seen to be connected and relevant to one another. As we have seen, recent developments in the field of sexuality and social work have suggested a broad range of shifts occurring, yet at times these seem disparate and characterized by events relevant to specific areas of practice (Dunk-West, Hafford-Letchfield, & Quinney 2009, Hafford-Letchfield 2008). Whilst sexuality may be aligned with love (Bauman 2004, Beck-Gernsheim 1999, Luhmann 1986) or intimacy (Giddens 1992), it has been equally used as a euphemism meaning sexual minorities (Dunk 2007). Sexual identity relates to the seemingly essentialist categories including lesbian, gay, bisexual as well as transgender, intersex, queer and questioning. These categories themselves, however, may bring with them uncertainty: viewed through a constructivist lens, queer may become a sensibility, a performative dimension of identity or a way of seeing the world (Seidman 1995). Viewed categorically, however these identities represent important markers of self-representation, vital for not only selfhood but for the basis upon which injustice on the grounds of sexual identity may be fought. The dualist importance of both individual subjectivity as well as social visibility resonate through definitions relating to sexuality and can be seen in the varied approaches this edited collection represents.

Sexuality and social work have a complex history that is impossible to discern without an awareness of the epistemological grounding of sexuality and its relationship to social work as a whole. Put simply this means that in order to understand the context in which sexuality is played out in social work, we need to be aware of wider political, social and interpersonal shifts that ripple through the profession of social work. The ways these broader changes are realized are manifold but include the very nature and timing of policies and practices that in turn define social work. In not only seeing sexuality as part of our individual psyches and bodies, but broadening our examination to societal attitudes and values, we can see that as attitudes towards sexuality have changed so too has social work experienced sexuality in differing manifestations.

The varied and diverse feminist and queer movements that have endured throughout the past four decades have, amongst both broad and specific contributions to political and social spheres, ostensibly destabilized traditional norms and values. This has meant that we can now speak about sexuality in a way that is different from previous generations. The sexual dimension to human experience has taken on new meanings and associations: reasons for engaging in sexual behaviour are varied and sex is no longer seen as necessarily having to occur within monogamous, heterosexual relationships for the purpose of procreation. The association of pleasure with sexual activity has signalled a major shift away from traditional norms and roles, including in particular, women's roles (Giddens 1992) and shifts in family relationships. Changes in partnering patterns and the very format of intimate relationships have been realized throughout social work settings in which professionals work with couples and individuals such as in children's and adults' services. These changes have been theorized in the social work literature associated with family relationships (Hicks 2005) and, within this book, are explored in the different chapters on foster care, adoption and lesbian parenting.

Aside from shifts in family relationships, the rise of therapeutic culture (Furedi 2004) that has coincided with recent social shifts (Lasch 1979, Reiff 1966) has transformed sexuality and sexual identity into the domain of expert knowledge. Indeed, Freud's sexuality (Freud 1905/1953) attests to a legacy in which the sexual self is laden with meaning and represents internalized struggles and tensions. Childhood experiences are linked to sexual '… psychical phenomena that we come across later in adult erotic life – such as fixation to particular objects, jealousy and so on' (Freud 1905/1953:159). Though Freudian and more contemporary psychoanalytic characterizations of sexuality remain ubiquitous in modern day helping professions and popular culture alike, critiques of this tradition remain. Indeed feminist scholars in the 1970s (Chodorow 1972, Firestone 1970, Millett 1970, Mitchell 1974) critiqued Freud's notion of sexuality on the grounds that masculine traits were depicted as overwhelmingly dominant over women's. Yet what we may draw from psychoanalytic approaches is that they place sexuality at the individual level. Subjective thoughts, actions and interactions are of interest over and above social mores and values. In social work we can see the association of sexuality with expert knowledge through the splintering of specialized services for dealing with issues relating to the intimate realm. With the association of sexuality with the individual sphere, social work practice has focussed on client sexuality, for example, when it has been a specific issue for a specific client. For example, a same-sex attracted young person may be involved with a social worker because of concerns for their safety due to homophobic attacks at school. Conversations about the young person's sexuality and sexual identity would occur in the context of their safety, and yet represent an individual focus because such conversations about sexuality and identity may not be seen to be relevant for a heterosexual identifying young person. Specialized services in sexual health, such as those provided in GUM (genitourinary medicine) clinics provide one to one medical and professional services. Again, these reflect the association of an individualized sexuality with expert knowledge and services. Some of these specific issues are discussed in this book and the importance of providing safe environments (for women for example) within mental health services. Two chapters are devoted to thinking through some of the potential harm that can occur where social work has not been clear about what sexual activity is acceptable and what constitutes abuse. Both chapters provide telling descriptions of contemporary mental health systems in which expert knowledge can curtail freedom of sexuality and sexual identity.

Counter to these subjective and intra-psychic notions of sexuality, Foucault's (Foucault 1978) investigation of sexuality acts to radically destabilize its psychoanalytic notions. Mostly relegated to considerations named as post structural, approaches that seek to disrupt firmly held ideas about sexuality such as those advanced by Foucault (Foucault 1978) and others, for example, within queer theory (Butler 1990, 1993), have been highly influential in scholarly thinking about the nature of sexuality. These traditions rely upon the notion of constructionism: sexuality is seen as 'made'. Making sexuality involves many differing forces and shifts which all come together to form unique and specific social conditions, which are in turn experienced by individuals. For Foucault, this making occurs at the social level, whereas for Butler it is within individual bounds that we may subvert and re-make the seemingly innate categories of gender and sexuality. In social work this means a re-orientation towards the social sphere – for it is within society that sexuality and sexual identities are 'made'. Narrative therapy is one of the orientations that social work has embraced, particularly for therapeutic work, and is aligned with constructivist traditions. Notably, narrative approaches see '… people as the experts in their own lives' (Morgan 2000:2) and people therefore 'make' their identities, including their sexual selves.

On the one hand we have innate sexuality that is assigned to individual psyches and bodily sensations and on the other we are presented with sexuality as a social and individual invention. Rather than following a linear trajectory, each of these traditions, that is, psychoanalytic and post structural, can be seen to co-exist in the broadly-based contemporary social work literature while also being realized distinctively throughout social work practice. For example, there has been a steady stream of research and scholarship into sexual behaviour which can be ontologically linked to traditions that see sexuality as innate to human nature generally. Sexual health, for example, is a field in which medical knowledge dominates (for example, see these influential earlier works: Kinsey 1948, 1953, Kraft-Ebing 1965, Masters & Johnson 1966, 1992). Sexual health research into, for example, HIV, Hepatitis C and other sexually transmissible infections, primarily relates to establishing modes of transmission by examining sexual behaviour. Thus, discourses of risk (Harvey, Hayen, & Eyeson-Annan 2003, Ryan 2005) feature heavily within such a paradigm (for more about risk, see Beck 1992, 1999). Though social work has traditionally engaged in both therapeutic culture as well as medical discourses (for example, consider the burgeoning field of addiction), the profession also has a strong tradition of sociological analyses involving broader social structures and the social meanings that individuals bring to their worlds. To this end, three chapters in this book speak to sexuality as it relates to identity by looking at identity from both organizational and individual perspectives. In summary, the chapters in this edited book are all written by women who have either a specific research or practice interest within the wide arena of sexuality and sexual identity, and the following synopsis we hope will guide your further reading.

In Chapter One, Hafford-Letchfield explores the tensions and complexities inherent in identity in terms of gender and sexuality within organizational contexts. Drawing from recent literature and research relating to organizations and sexuality and gender and how these are subsequently 'enacted' in the workplace, this chapter highlights the importance of awareness in challenging and subverting dominant biases relating to both sexuality and gender. This paints a particularly complex and contradictory picture of what progress is actually being made towards gender and sexual equality and highlights the more subtle practices embedded within social work's core processes and activities. Hafford-Letchfield calls for increased reflexivity in order to negotiate boundaries within such an institutionalized script and makes some tentative recommendations about what can be done to deconstruct and challenge some of these discursive practices.

Chapter Two brings us Sarah Carr's user perspective on '"A Chance to Cut is a Chance to Cure": Self-harm and Self-protection – a Gay Perspective', which incorporates medicalized and sociological knowledge into a powerful and moving reflective piece. In her chapter Carr critically examines the placement of self-harm within mental health discourse. She concludes with a consideration of the 'personalization' agenda and how lesbian, gay and bisexual people might be best supported within this framework. Carr's chapter provides telling descriptions of contemporary mental health systems in which expert knowledge can curtail freedom of sexuality and sexual identity. We are reminded that whilst it may be tempting to cast lesbian and gay sexual identities being associated with mental illness as a quirk of history, sexuality and expert knowledge retain their associations to one another in contemporary social work settings. Carr's perspective is a unique one but can be added to the growing body of user-generated knowledge on this under theorized topic.

Chapter Three is the first of two chapters which address the topics of age and sexuality. Age is a growing area of awareness in diversity studies and sexuality and in this chapter Rhiannon Jones documents her research journey and some early findings from her PhD study into older women's sexualities. Jones reflects upon the challenges posed in researching older women's sexuality, sexual desire and activity, which continues at best to be marginalized and at worst invisible. She explores and analyses the myriad of methodological considerations vital to such research. Participants' views about the research method itself enable a deeper appreciation of not only how to research with older people about sexuality but what questions ought to be being empirically defined and explored. Jones concludes that for both research and social work practice, engaging with older people around issues of sexuality is necessary in order to challenge their exclusion. The centrality of sexuality to identity, sense of self and personhood only makes it even more urgent that the experiences and voices of older people are heard.

In Chapter Four Michelle Brown and Priscilla Dunk-West turn the focus on to young women's sexualities. Like older women's sexualities, Brown and Dunk-West highlight the social milieus in which young people's sexualities are located and the subsequent complexities that are associated with the social and subjective spheres of experience. An auto-ethnographic methodology was used to elicit material for this chapter. Though co-written, material has been drawn from Michelle Brown's practice in sexual health and is therefore presented as a first person, reflective account. What we learn is that the placement of pleasure within sexual health discourses is one that is problematic and often at odds with the long list of issues the sexual health worker is charged with tackling. Brown and Dunk-West also reflect on what gets in the way of promoting pleasure as a legitimate and sometimes political aspect to sexuality. The chapter argues that the 'business' of sexual health is controlled by various pressures including the need to reduce sexually transmissible infections and unplanned pregnancies. Brown and Dunk-West outline how pleasure ought to fit in with the concept of sexuality as well as within educational work in sexual health. Both Jones and Brown and Dunk-West in chapters three and four argue for social work approaches that take into account subjective experiences of sexuality yet demonstrate that social and subjective constructions of age are relevant to the work.

Chapter Five by Anna Fairtlough provides us with an opportunity to hear first hand from young people who grew up with a lesbian or gay parent, and is one of three chapters in this text which discusses ideological and practice shifts to partnering patterns and the very format of intimate relationships. These have been realized throughout social work services in which professionals work with couples and individuals such as in children's and adults' services. These changes have already been theorized in social work literature associated with family relationships (Hicks 2005). In this chapter Fairtlough reports on a qualitative content analysis of accounts published in collected anthologies and magazines, by young people of having a lesbian or gay parent. Drawing from life story approaches, she facilitates our ability to better hear from this 'hidden population' of young people. Fairtlough's chapter powerfully highlights the structural homophobia inherent in our culture and in the environment within which the young people lived. The chapter concludes with pertinent considerations of the implications for practice in the United Kingdom.

Chapter Six by Jeanette Copperman challenges us yet again with regard to sexuality and mental health. She brings to our sharp attention a relatively unknown, little publicized, but very significant public inquiry – the Kerr/Haslam inquiry – into two consultant psychiatrists convicted of sexual abuse against vulnerable female patients over a twenty year period. Through the eyes of this inquiry, Copperman investigates the abuse of power within mental health services. It is through the analysis of the Kerr/Haslam inquiry that she highlights a number of key themes. Firstly, she illustrates how professionals colluded to hide abuse and the influence of organizational culture in abusive settings; and secondly, she reflects on organizational gender relations in the context of power inequalities. Given that social work is often in the eyes of the media, Copperman examines the professional, public and media responses to Kerr/Haslam within discourses about serious case reviews.

In Chapter Seven, Helen Cosis Brown offers us yet another perspective on family relationships and sexual identity through the analysis of foster care and parenting assessment practice. Cosis Brown draws on the findings of an explorative qualitative study into the content and quality of the assessments of lesbian and gay men prospective foster carers. She uses an historical approach by looking back at key changes to the legislative framework, policy, and research relevant to this area of social work practice. Cosis Brown critically explores the relationship and interesting position that social work has to broader social shifts in the creation of lesbian and gay families. She investigates how these are realized through the practice of assessment and the importance of gaining confidence and support to deflect society's continuing ambivalence, particularly in light of the Wakefield enquiry.

Chapter Eight shifts from a focus on sexual minorities to considering heterosexuality. In 'What is Personal? Reflecting on Heterosexuality', Joy Trotter uses focused reflection to examine this under-theorized area of inquiry in social work. The over-reliance on theoretical work about lesbian, gay, bisexual and transgender sexualities is shown to have meant that heterosexuality has been without a critical lens in social work theory. Trotter argues for the unravelling of some of the complexities involved in this area of human experience and differing epistemologies. Using the three areas of emotions, relationships and identities, Trotter traces the way sexual identity has been treated within social work contexts. The chapter concludes with a personal reflection that calls for feminist understandings of heterosexuality as well as openness and veracity in policy and practice. Trotter reasserts the feminist notion that personal experience is a relevant and valid form of knowledge.

In Chapter Nine, Christine Cocker explores sexual identity and adoption, offering us yet another perspective on family relationships, but this time from adopters' perspectives. Her chapter entitled 'Sexuality before Ability? The Assessment of Lesbians as Adopters', reports on an under researched area of empirical knowledge. There is little known about the efficacy of the adoption assessment experiences of lesbians who have adopted children. Drawing on her own interview data, Cocker's chapter provides in depth accounts in which lesbian adopters describe their experience of the assessment process and how the adoption assessment experience prepared them to make decisions about adoptions. Particularly of interest is her exploration of how issues specific to the sexual identities of the adopters were raised and discussed by the social workers assessing them and the quality and complexity of practice in this area.

Chapter Ten reminds us that one of the benefits in seeing sexuality as being constructed individually is that it enables diversity to be realized. Striving towards deeper approaches to learning about sexuality inevitably raises a gamut of complexities around which pedagogical practices are useful in social work education. Aymer and Patni provide a unique analysis of diversity including discussions about culture and race, gender, sexual identity and religion, rarely found in the social work education literature. Their discussion is oriented around pedagogical considerations of diversity and, importantly, the chapter represents a move toward critical discussion of the disjunct between individualized notions of selfhood and structural considerations for socially just inclusion. They assert that challenging our own and others religions and cultures should be part and parcel of social work education and the important contribution of such learning to developing a professional identity needs to be more fully realized. This requires conscious effort from the different partners involved as well as the utilization of different theoretical arguments as a means of embracing difference and challenging oppressive structures combined with critical reflection.

Finally in Chapter Eleven, Dunk-West argues that we need to reconceptualize the way we think about identity in social work in order to accommodate the creative and complex ways individuals construct their sexualities. Reporting on the findings from a qualitative study in which thirty participants with 'non problematic sexuality' were interviewed about their sexual selves, Dunk-West asks whether it is possible to separate out our sexuality from a broader identity into what she terms the 'de-differentiated self'. Theorizing identity as 'de-differentiated' has implications for social work and ultimately it is argued that social work ought to rethink some of the existing ways of communicating and recording client information, as it is only through appreciating the historical and social embeddedness of identity that we may seek to better understand subjectivity.

When seen as a whole, the chapters contained within *Sexual Identities and Sexuality in Social Work* represent a telling snapshot of current scholarship and movements within the broad sphere of social work and sexuality. They make reference to the influences of modernist constructions of sexuality alongside more post structural visions of the sexual subject and represent the latest in research and scholarship in this important area. This is, of course, by no means a complete collection as there are many more topics and issues beyond the scope of this text and to which references are made within the different chapters. The contributions contained in this collection encourage thinking and debate: both broadly as well as within specifically defined areas of social work, both of which are crucial to continued scholarship, practice and research in sexuality within the complex setting of social work in contemporary times. We hope you enjoy them.

References

Bauman, Z. 2004. *Liquid Love: On the Frailty of Human Bonds*. Cambridge: Polity Press.

Beck-Gernsheim, E. 1999. On the Way to a Post-Familial Family: From a Community of Need to Elective Affinities, in *Love and Eroticism*, edited by M. Featherstone. London: Sage.

Beck, U. 1992. *Risk Society*. London: Sage.

Beck, U. 1999. *World Risk Society*. Cambridge: Polity Press.

Butler, J. 1990. *Gender Trouble: Feminism and the Subversion of Identity*. New York: Routledge.

Butler, J. 1993. *Bodies that Matter: On the Discursive Limits of 'Sex'*. London: Routledge.

Chodorow, N. 1972. *Women and Madness*. New York: Doubleday.

Dunk-West, P., Hafford-Letchfield, T. & Quinney, A. 2009. Editorial: practice, sexuality and gender: intersections in social work. *Practice: Social Work in Action*, 21(1), 1–3.

Dunk, P. 2007. Everyday sexuality and social work: locating sexuality in professional practice and education. *Social Work & Society*, 5(2), 135–142.

Eraut, M. 1994. *Developing Professional Knowledge and Competence*. London and New York: Routledge Falmer.

Firestone, S. 1970. *The Dialectic of Sex: The Case for Feminist Revolution*. New York: Bantam Books.

Foucault, M. 1978. *The History of Sexuality: Volume One, The Will to Knowledge*. London: Penguin Books.

Freud, S. 1905/1953. Three Essays on the Theory of Sexuality (J. Strachey, Trans.) *Complete Psychological Works*. London: Hogarth Press, 125–243.

Furedi, F. 2004. *Therapy Culture: Cultivating Vulnerability in an Uncertain Age*. London: Routledge.

Giddens, A. 1992. *The Transformation of Intimacy: Sexuality, Love and Eroticism in Modern Societies*. Stanford: Stanford University Press.

Hafford-Letchfield, T. 2008. What's love got to do with it? Developing supportive practices for the expression of sexuality, sexual identity and the intimacy needs of older people. *Journal of Care Services Management*, 2(4), 389–405.

Harvey, L., Hayen, A. & Eyeson-Annan, M. 2003. *Continuous NSW Health Survey: Quarterly Report on Health Status, Health Behaviours, and Risk Factors*. New South Wales: New South Wales Public Health Bulletin.

Hicks, S. 2005. Is gay parenting bad for kids? Responding to the 'very idea of difference' in research on lesbian and gay parents. *Sexualities*, 8(2), 153–168.

Kinsey, A.C. 1948. *Sexual Behavior in the Human Male*. Philadelphia: Saunders.

Kinsey, A.C. 1953. *Sexual Behavior in the Human Female*. Philadelphia: Saunders.

Kraft-Ebing, R. v.1965. *Psychopathia Sexualis*. New York: Putnam.

Lasch, C. 1979. *The Culture of Narcissism: American Life in an Age of Diminishing Expectations*. New York: WW Norton.

Lewis, J. 2003. 'The Contribution of Research Findings to Practice Change'. Edited by J. Henderson & D. Atkinson, *Managing Care in Context*. London: Routledge.

Luhmann, N. 1986. *Love as Passion: The Codification of Intimacy*. Cambridge: Harvard University Press.

Masters, W. & Johnson, V. 1966. *Human Sexual Response*. Boston: Little Brown.

Masters, W. & Johnson, V. 1992. *Heterosexuality*. London: HarperCollins Publishers.

Millett, K. 1970. *Sexual Politics*. New York: Doubleday.

Mitchell, J. 1974. *Psychoanalysis and Feminism*. New York: Pantheon Books.

Morgan, A. 2000. *What is Narrative Therapy?* Adelaide: Dulwich Centre Publications.

Reiff, P. 1966. *The Triumph of the Therapeutic: Uses of Faith after Freud*. New York: Harper and Row.

Ryan, A. 2005. From Dangerous Sexualities to Risky Sex: Regulating Sexuality in the name of Public Health, in *Perspectives in Human Sexuality*, edited by G. Hawkes & J.G. Scott. South Melbourne: Oxford University Press, 203–216.

Seidman, S. 1995. Deconstructing Queer Theory or the Under-theorization of the Social and the Ethical, in *Social Postmodernism: Beyond Identity Politics*, edited by L. Nicholson & S. Seidman. Cambridge: Cambridge University Press, 116–141.

Chapter 1

Sexuality and Women in Care Organizations: Negotiating Boundaries within a Gendered Cultural Script

Trish Hafford-Letchfield

Introduction

Mainstream research, education and practice in management and organizations in social work have not been strong on gender and sexuality and any specific analysis is far from being explicit and well established. This chapter therefore takes a closer look at the contradictory and paradoxical nature of gendered selves and sexual identities in those public sector organizations delivering care services. Research into gender issues in care organizations has historically been influenced by the feminist movement and by a number of critical studies on social issues where gender as a biological fixed entity has been analysed for its social, historical, economic and political constructions (Dominelli 2002, Orme 1998, White 2006). Most of this has focussed on service user perspectives and their experiences and the nature of relationships between social workers and service users. Despite these theoretical developments, gender and gender powered relations within social care organizations themselves have been less of a concern. This is despite the fact that gender and sexuality issues remain defining features in most social care organizations: for example in gendered patterns of hierarchy; occupational segregation; the predominance of heterosexuality; harassment and discrimination and in the questioning of work–life balance, particularly in relation to family responsibilities. These are in turn defined by and instrumental in reproducing social relations of age, class, disability, culture and ethnicity.

Similarly, major changes in the United Kingdom legislative framework to promote the rights of lesbians and gay men have challenged and continue to challenge long-standing heteronormative and heterosexist frames of reference in both social work practice and professional education and the way these are organized. Numerous developments in legislation and rights to promote sexuality within particular areas such as employment, crime, civil partnership and family law have gone some way to transforming the everyday lives and experiences of lesbian, gay and bisexual people (Cocker and Hafford-Letchfield 2010). However, in the absence of any current systematic approach to addressing sexuality issues in social work, there are implications for its increased visibility and the complexity of managing identities within the current dynamic and changing social environment in which care organizations operate.

Theoretically, a move towards more pluralist approaches within the post structuralist and post modernist turns has also given rise to the intersection of gender and sexuality with other multiple social divisions and differences. Those 'third wave' feminists have critically questioned the notion of coherent identities and view freedom as resistance to categorization or identity (Mann and Huffman 2004). Evolving discourses frame and determine social knowledge and our subsequent understanding of power as well as about the concentration of power in relation to the nature of personal identity and organizational life. These continue to carry gendered meanings and reinforce gender inequalities (Foucault 1977, Broadbridge and Hearn 2008). Globalization and individualization, together with increasingly individualized consumer cultures within modernization of care services (Clarke 2004) and more recently the UK governments 'transformation' agenda (Department of Health 2008) have demanded continuous innovation and performance improvement in all aspects of social care. Within this context we face a particularly complex and contradictory picture of what progress is actually being made towards gender and sexual equality.

This chapter will argue that whilst a number of gains have been achieved, if left critically unexamined, sexism, heterosexism and gender biases will continue as more subtle practices embedded within social work's core processes and activities. This requires increased reflexivity in order to negotiate boundaries within such an institutionalized cultural script (Martin 2003). By reviewing some of the literature and research on gender and sexuality within organizations in social work and social care, this chapter intends to elaborate on the range of ways that gender and sexuality are enacted, sustained and generated across the structures and practices of organizational life. It reviews some of the broader key discourses when thinking about the relationships between gender, sexuality and organizations within social care. Some tentative recommendations will be made about what women themselves can do, what care organizations can do and how current discursive practice in relation to gender and sexuality within the organization might be deconstructed and challenged.

Gender, sexuality and social work – a brief historical perspective

The meaning of gender and sexuality in social work has changed over time and is by its very nature, politically and socially constructed. A number of debates and movements arising from feminist activism from the 1970s have supported women's rights both in the workplace and in service provision giving rise to positive responses through legislation, social policy, human resource developments and service delivery (Dominelli and McLeod 1989). Public concern and recognition of issues such as sexual harassment, sexual abuse and examination of opportunities for women in relation to promoting fairness in career progression and in exercising their rights are examples of evidence of positive responses to these issues (White 2006).

Orme (2009:69–71), who has contributed extensively to the literature in this area, identifies three strands of feminist social work informed by and responsive to developments in feminist thinking. Firstly she highlights the synergies between feminism and social work based on shared values where the latter has used categories such as race, gender and class to legitimize action against oppression. Feminist social work has strived to work with women to raise consciousness but also considers subjectivity of the individual, their sense of self and ways of understanding their relationship within the world. The ethos of this relationship enables women to utilize their strengths and abilities as both a resource and means of exercising their rights (Hanmer and Statham 1999). For example, increased levels of awareness and developments in responses to domestic violence over the last decade are largely due to the determined efforts of women's organizations forcing domestic violence from the margin to the mainstream (Blyth 2005). The subsequent emergence of multi-agency domestic violence fora has encouraged professionals from different disciplines not to think in boxes but to understand the overlap between different forms of oppression. These have proved essential not just in understanding safeguarding implications within family social work but in making connections with other types of abuse in vulnerable adults (Department of Health 2000). Secondly, Orme refers to 'prescriptions for practice with women' by utilizing commonalities and differences to build a basis for which relationships can be built between women workers and service users. One critique of this approach is the potential homogenization of the category of 'woman'. The sustainability of this position is questionable on the basis that it does not fully acknowledge the presence of power. How it is grounded in the realities of practice particularly for providers of state services within a statutory context is also questionable (Hale 1984, White 2006). Thirdly, Orme cites the importance of understanding gender dimensions of social work by adopting feminist theory to explore the impact of gender oppression on men and social work such as in the work done by Cree (2001).

Correll et al. (2007:1) define gender as:

> an institutionalized system of practices for constituting people as two different categories (men and women), and organizing relations of inequality based on this difference.

This definition captures several key features of contemporary views on gender. Gender is seen as a categorization process which starts on the basis of classification and differentiation and then applied to persons, activities, behaviours, jobs, tasks, objects and so on (Mathieu 2009).

In short there are many complications in conceptualizing gender and defining what it is. Whilst the nature of women's experiences and gender issues have been explored in much greater depth within a number of social science disciplines, the significance of gender and sexuality within many areas of social care have not. For example the implications for women within significant user groups such as older people (Maynard et al. 2008) and people with learning disabilities (Scior 2003) in all their diverse contexts remain relatively or at least inconsistently unexplored as care environments have developed. There has been some bringing together of issues in relation to gender and sexuality, for example, Brown and Cocker (2010) tell us that:

> The second wave of the women's movement ... brought together lesbian and feminist political discourses. It was within this area that much of the radical thinking about social work and feminism as well as social work with lesbians and gay men took place (Brown and Cocker 2011:8).

The rise of lesbian and gay political influences through activists and organizations within the UK Socialist movement, its Local Authorities, Councillors and Unions up to the 1980s had advanced the nature of much public sector thinking compared with later hostilities emanating from later Conservative Governments. Social work in the 1980s was one of the professions at the forefront of arguing for lesbian and gay equality as demonstrated through social work's involvement within trade union as well as labour and community activism (Brown 1998). However, looking at the changed landscape of social work from the 1990s towards the end of the first decade of the 21st century, many of its challenges lie in being compliant with legislative and policy requirements. The trend towards increased managerialism; bureau-professional regimes within specific configurations of structures, cultures, relationships and processes of organizational co-ordination (Clarke and Newman 1997) served to dampen the organizational base from which the women's movement and its supporters had operated. Substantial growth in legislation, policy and practice guidance and proceduralization has standardized many areas of social work practice in which organizational compliance has become a crucial and valued quality (Harlow 2004). More recent moves towards personalization and self-directed care (Department of Health 2008a) have been critiqued for the potential to take service users further away from any analysis of their structural, community and personal circumstances (Ferguson 2007). Any in-depth analysis of the causes of social problems, or service users' own narratives of their situation have become secondary to procedures, resource allocation and measurement of 'outcomes' (Hafford-Letchfield 2010). The individualization of service provision can further lead to the undermining of collective service provision (Ferguson, 2007). Hudson, writing more than two decades ago, still captures the issues relevant to contemporary social work's organizational structures and their influence.

In reality, the structure and control of social work reflects and reinforces broader social processes of male domination in our society. Feminism's central emphasis on women participating in the decisions affecting them (as consumers and as workers) and on creating decision-making structures which are non-hierarchical, very directly confronts the masculine organizational principles of social work agencies (Hudson 1985:640–641).

What does organisational theory tell us?

Organizations are embodied in their social contexts being both social places of organizing and social structuring of social relations. Their interrelationships are historically dynamic (Hearn and Parkin 2001). Classical theory and scientific management carry implicit and sometimes explicit conceptualizations of gender and sexuality where managerial practices spell out detailed statements on the way one is assumed to manage or be managed. Weberarian concepts of the bureaucratic organization (Weber 1947) tend to emphasize rationality or instrumentality rather than emotions whereas in practice, bureaucracies are often intensely emotional. The human relations school has been interpreted by Hearn and Parkin (2001) as an attempt by men not just to reorganize social relationships in organizations but to incorporate gendered and sexual relations in to organizational analysis. This is presented in an agendered and asexual way by using neutral language. Hearn and Parkin go as far to suggest that human relations theory has been used to legitimate increased managerial surveillance and control of workers, particularly women's emotional and even sexual lives.

Likewise the bringing of psychoanalytic insights from individual to group and organizational dynamics, such as those enshrined in the theoretical conceptions of the UK Tavistock Institute, has addressed the unconscious preoccupations of members of groups and organizations. These include unconscious sexual preoccupations and have contributed significantly to the government of subjectivity and social life (Hearn and Parkin 2001).

All of these theories have, albeit in different ways, contributed to the establishment of the system as the prime paradigm for the analysis of organizations. According to Hearn and Parkin (who have written extensively in the area of gender, sexuality and violence in organizations), the system can be used to obscure gender and sexuality. In another sense, it can also be used to perpetuate or justify the maintenance roles of women in lower organizational positions. Whichever way one looks at it, Hearn and Parkin suggest that organizational theories and analysis are more frequently concerned with human relations that express interpersonal and emotional relationships between its members rather than those social structural relations of power and dominance. Therefore the notion of organizational structure as an objective, empirical and genderless reality is itself a gendered notion. The range of empirical studies outlined in the unique text 'The Sexuality of Organizations' (Hearn et al. 1989) for example, highlights these interconnections of sexuality and power in organizations and the pervasiveness of the power of men, particularly heterosexual men.

Connecting gender and sexuality in social work organizations

There are gendered processes in sexuality, including the dominance of various forms of sexuality over others. On the face of it, sex and sexuality might appear to have little to do with social care management and organizations. One might even argue that the current bureaucratic and managerialist organization is predominantly viewed as sexless, emanating from its rational and objective character. Sexuality can also be understood as both a foundation of gender and a focused aspect of gender relations. A growing body of research however has promulgated theories on how heterosexuality is seen as the primary means by which both people and organizations are gendered and as a mechanism through which power is exercised within the organizational context (Gutek 1989, Brown 1995, Halford and Leonard 2001, Hicks 2008). By exploring aspects of communication, career development, self-presentation and relationships within organizations, a heterosexualised version of sexuality inflects organizational life at all levels with gendered consequences. Most organizations and managements reproduce dominant heterosexual norms, ideology and practices. One of the consequences of which is to render gay and lesbian issues 'problematic' where gay men and lesbian women are forced to 'manage' their sexuality in organizations, choosing whether to come out and how to manage this out identity (which is more than a one off event) or more commonly to hide their identity. Research commissioned by Stonewall in 2008 revealed the tensions and contradictions which exist for lesbian women at work. It suggested that often lesbian women think their gender is more of a barrier to success at work than their sexual orientation. Therefore, if they can hide the fact that they're gay, some feel it best to do just that. As one participant said, 'putting your hand up twice' can be difficult (Miles not dated:2). Participants felt that role models and openly gay women made a crucial difference to the confidence and profile of lesbians and bisexual women in the workplace, and wanted to see organizations involve them more in the development and its initiatives:

> As a woman you've already got one strike against you in terms of a diversity box that you check. As a lesbian that's the second one as well. If you're an ethnic minority lesbian then you've got three. As a woman and as an ethnic minority you can't hide that, but there's no reason to foreground the fact you're gay as well. People feel that it's hard enough (quoted research participant in Miles, not dated:7).

Like monitoring established in other areas of diversity, effective monitoring of sexual orientation can be an important tool for employers to measure performance and make improvements to the working environment. This however is not an exercise that can succeed in isolation. It highlights differences between groups, such as minority status or staff from particular teams or grades, in terms of productivity, satisfaction and progression (Stonewall not dated).

Indeed (hetero)sexual arrangements in private domains generally provide the base infrastructure for organizations and management, principally through women's associated unpaid reproductive labour (Broadbridge and Hearn 2008). One might think that there would tend to be more sensitivity or at least tolerance within social work environments to these complexities. Whilst legislative changes may have, in turn, transformed the current context for social work practice with lesbians and gay men, challenges for practice remain as this will only 'be as effective as the practitioners and managers responsible for its implementation' (Dugmore and Cocker 2008:166). Brown and Cocker (2010:9) are broadly optimistic about the effect of recent protective legislation:

> [. . .] experiences of related struggles for equality, such as women's emancipation and race equality, would suggest that the journey ... has only really just begun.

However, according to Jeyasingham, 'There are plenty of examples of "continuing ignorance"'. (Jeyasingham 2008). One example is illustrated in the prevalence of sexual banter in day centres and care homes (Bauer and Geront 1999) and in everyday sexualized forms of communication; a jolly cheerful sort of sexuality which hints at constant availability, in which both men and women have to collude (Halford and Leonard 2001:157).

Women in management – opportunities for change?

Gendered division of labour in management within social care illustrates itself through exclusions and exclusion, and specialisation in particular forms of formal and informal labour with vertical and horizontal divisions in organizations and management (Broadbridge and Hearn 2008:541). Discourses about women managers in social care organizations construct women within a subordination relationship which automatically devalues everything that can be attributed to women (Gherardi 1994). On the other hand, women who 'reach the top' of an organization's hierarchy are then often desexualized or seen as 'career women'.

The woman who adopts a masculine style and behaviour is perceived as having been incorporated and criticized for assuming the status of an honorary man, while the woman who retains caring or service orientation risks being criticized for failing to conform to the models expected of a manager (Foster 1999).

Therefore, women's relational style can both help and hinder their effectiveness as leaders. A study of how women 'learn' to become managers undertaken by Bryans and Mavin (2003:129) demonstrated that this involves a complex combination of factors. They refer to the perception of women's personalities, their value systems, their experiences and the culture and interventions of the organizations within which they worked. Learning to 'become' a manager for participants in Bryans and Mavins' study revealed a story of change where a key issue centred on the woman's decision to change themselves or to change the management practice in their organizations. Reflecting on this (untypical) research within the management literature and particularly in the social work management literature, it appears that encouraging the narratives of women opens up more space for contestation and resistance. Greater insights are needed to provide more fluid definitions of different relationships at work whereby women can mobilize power to construct *themselves* within organizations, rather than be constructed by them.

Managerial ideologies and organizational mechanisms to enhance efficiency, accountability and competition have dominated and transformed the landscape for organizing and delivering social care (Clarke and Newman 1997). There is some evidence that these developments have actually reinforced some issues around inequality (White 2006, Ferguson 2007). Despite a number of aspirational system-wide standards for avoiding discrimination, promoting dignity and person-centred, individualized care within public policy relating to care (HM Government et al. 2006, Department of Health 2007, 2008, 2008a) policy in relation to gender and sexuality issues is rarely made explicit or has a tendency to be cast as neutral and uncontentious (Harlow 2003, Cocker and Hafford-Letchfield 2010). However, extensive research into front line social work reveals how restructuring has resulted in the de-skilling and intensification of practice and in low morale for many front line workers (Morrison 2007, Children's Workforce Development Council 2006). Whilst there has been a continuous stream of helpful insights drawn from the critical literature on management (Clarke 2004; Hafford-Letchfield et al. 2008, Lawler and Bilson 2010) a few studies (Maddock 1999, Healy 2002, and Aronson and Smith 2009) have focused on the experiences of those who manage social and community services. These have highlighted how managers, particularly women managers might distance themselves from managerialist practices or develop resistance to find more participatory opportunities for staff and service users. In a qualitative study of Canadian women managers, Aronson and Smith (2009) discerned two broad strategies deployed by women to develop the critical consciousness of those they managed. These included; efforts to expand entitlements to service users increasingly excluded from public support and; efforts to politicize and expand the scope of practice in their organizations by sustaining advocacy in their work and; embedding sophisticated knowledge of institutional politics and enormous skill in using language to expand, deepen practice and developing the critical consciousness of those they managed:

> We're able to mediate everybody coming together mostly on that 'this would be helpful for women' ... as long as you'd speak about 'policy development', 'planning'. I mean who could say no to that right? ... I mean municipalities and certainly policy people in the government will always say; oh yes we need to 'coordinate' you know? So we played up to that stuff (participant quoted in Aronson and Smith 2009:14).

The above quote illustrates the internalization of gendered divisions of authority in management, both formal and informal, and the way in which women and men may be valued differentially in terms of both formal authority, by virtue of their post and positions and informal authority from their status and standing in the organization.

Leadership

Leadership is a gendered concept and as suggested earlier is applied within a social context itself that is gendered (Yoder 2001). These understandings are crucial as leadership is cited as the key to delivering the UK Government's vision of quality services and highlights the specific role of managers in shaping and changing services (Department for Education and Skills 2006, Department of Health 2008, Department for Children, Schools and Families 2009). The importance of effective leadership and management in social work is emphasized in the context of recent policy and practice developments in the UK and elsewhere, with frequent reference to the relationship between 'transforming services' and 'effective leadership' (Department of Health 2008). Critical markers for evaluating the gender congeniality of the social context in which leadership is embedded include group composition, the gender-typing of the task, valuing task performance over all other outcomes, and power emphases (Yoder 2001). Yoder proposes a gender sensitive model where exploring leader effectiveness recognizes both the gender of the leader and the gender congeniality of the context in which the leader operates. The leadership literature is also highly masculinized by drawing on stereotypical skills evaluated for goal attainment within a hierarchical organization where power bases operate. Models of transformation and charismatic leadership emphasize influence rather than power, and empowerment of self and others such as concepts of distributed leadership which are largely equated with team work and collaboration (Hafford-Letchfield et al. 2008). Highlighting the gendered stereotyping of leaders, Eagly and Carly (2007) likewise give examples of everyday descriptions used to describe leaders as 'competitive', 'political', 'ambitious', 'driven', 'social', 'tough', 'task focused', 'instrumental', 'passionate' and 'committed'. These are seen as positive attributes for men but seen as negative for women. Mavin (2009) distinguishes these from communal behaviours which are more helpful, sympathetic, empathetic and compassionate and highly valued in traditional social work practice with more agentic behaviours, such as 'assertive', 'controlled', 'determined', 'self-reliant', 'independent' and 'individualistic'. The latter agentic behaviours are automatically assumed as resulting in effective leadership, whereas communal behaviours are not (Eagly and Carly 2007). This is despite the fact that women who display agentic behaviours are likely to jolt assumptions about how they should behave thereby highlighting the different expectations of how men and women can vent emotions. For example, traditional gendered emotion behaviours include mothering, nurturing and caring roles, supporting and developing others and resolving conflict. According to Mavin (2001) a woman's success as a leader therefore depends on how well or how poorly she navigates her way through her sexual stereotype and her work competence and how men and women judge that balancing act.

In summary, any critical analysis of gender and sexuality within social care organizations entails looking beyond and deconstructing the obvious, and the dominant taken-for-granted perspectives by which organizations are constructed and analysed. In doing so, one is shifting to the sub-texts of organizations such as gender, sexuality and the manifest forms of processes around these. According to Halford and Leonard (2001:26), in reviewing theoretical perspectives, the key to achieving a more integrated understanding of the relations between gender, sexuality and organizations lies in focusing attention on the question of 'power' as the lynchpin on which power is seen to flourish. The systematization of power relations between members in an organization enables organizational power to strengthen its position around gender and sexuality and vice versa, so that these then come to characterize some forms of organizational power.

Social theory and changing theorizations of gender and sexuality

The performative nature of gender has been broadly adopted within feminist and gender studies based mainly on the work by Judith Butler (1990), but has the potential to be applied to studies of gender in work, organization and management (Mathieu 2009). Discursive knowledge of the social systems we participate in (referred to as 'discursive penetration' by Giddens 1979:5) and being able to permeate between different types of knowledge enhances the potential for discursive articulation (Mathieu 2009). Mathieu talks about the move by recent feminist research away from intentionality or purposive action as the primary base for discrimination and sex inequality to what she terms as an approach based on 'non conscious cognitive processes' (2009:255). This performative-practice approach suggests that sexism and gender bias are more subtly constituted through non-reflexive practices which are rarely recognized or condemned, and form part of the broad institutionalized cultural scripts we follow (Martin 2006:255). Gender researchers in organizations contend that gender is a central feature of organizational life and deeply implicated in core processes and activities such as motivation, decision making, culture, identity and strategy. Research done by Martin (2006) illustrates how the practice of gender in workplaces is carried. She used vignettes of contextual, interactive gender performances, often entailing discursive inquiry or challenges. From this research she was able to distinguish between gendered practices and the practising of gender. Gendered practices, according to Martin (2003) are culturally available, appropriate, and usually unquestioned options that can be used by persons in particular positions in particular situations. Practising gender is the way in which such options or alternative activities are enacted or performed.

In this sense, performing masculinity (or behaving like a man) forsaking family and personal life, displaying assertiveness and risk-taking is paradigmatic. Where performances cannot be comfortably or skilfully deployed, there can be a downplaying or playing submissive to gain trust and acceptance. Alternatively, one can lead 'masculine' lives by downplaying the importance of family or personal lives (Mathieu 2009).

From a post structuralist perspective, discourses such as those of gender and sexuality within organizations are understood as having fluidity of meaning while power is understood as being dispersed between individuals, sometimes regardless of their formal structural position (Halford and Leonard 2001). This offers possibilities for contestation, transformation within any discursive situation. Whilst structural disadvantages shape the work experiences of many women, there are strategies of power and resistance open to them by resisting the dominant discourses by which their sexuality and identities are constructed within organizations.

Gendered assumptions about women in social work organizations – workforce issues

The association of management with the authority of position and social work with the authority of expertise fits neatly with the essentially gendered nature of the presentations of the occupations themselves and the anticipated gender of the occupants of the respective roles (Foster 1999). The position of women in the traditional professions is assumed to be relatively unproblematic since they 'fit very well 'with the attributes expected for the work carried out. The valuing of organizations and management themselves over that work takes place in more private domains for example in the valuing of men's work over women's (Broadbridge and Hearn 2008). Issues around integration and conflicting values between professions have further weakened attention to gender and sexuality, for example within medical models of care. There are many documented gendered relations of organizational participants to domestic and related responsibilities (Women's National Commission 2009). Women typically continue to carry the double burden of childcare and unpaid domestic work, and even a triple burden of care for dependents, including parents, older people and people with disabilities (Manthorpe 2003). Gendered assumptions about women's capacities to undertake endless quantities of caring labour uneasily inhabit a complicated mix of exploitation, ethical human behaviour, professional identity, and individual resistance against employers, the state and a wider, uncaring society (Baines 2004). Further, it is difficult to delineate these 'naturalized' notions of caring from professional caring skills. Notions of vocation, professional obligation, and duty and where these overlap, make social care workers an easy target for the sector-wide imperative to expand unwaged work (Baines 2004).

Ferguson (2007) highlights this potential in his critique of personalization in the UK government's 'Transformation' agenda:

> Concerns about the conditions (or lack of conditions) on which personal assistants for the employment of whom direct payments are commonly used were being hired. None of these criticisms is an argument against the use of direct payments per se but they do point to the need for greater discussion amongst service users, social work and health professionals and trade union activists to ensure that the legitimate desire of adults who require social care services for greater

independence is not exploited by governments intent on promoting increased privatization of services under the banner of 'welfare reform' (2007:398).

It is well known that the social care workforce is gender biased, with women forming eighty-four percent of the workforce. There are currently no formal requirements for monitoring of Lesbian, Gay, Bisexual or Transgendered populations in the workforce despite many imperatives to do so (Equality Commission 2009). Employers in England for example, completing the National Minimum Data Set (Skills for Care 2008) indicated that amongst employees where gender was recorded, eighty-four percent are female and sixteen percent are male. Part time workers within homecare showing within workforce data as having the highest turnover rate of the care sectors at nearly twenty-five per cent with an average of £6.80 pay per hour (Skills for Care 2008). The percentage of women is highest amongst Local Authorities (eighty-six percent) and lowest amongst the voluntary sector (eighty-one percent), (Hussein 2009). Women working in social care are also significantly older than men, with a median age of forty-three years. Different characteristics such as age, ethnicity and gender vary by different job roles grouped as; direct care workers, managers, supervisors, professionals and other workers. So for example, within direct care, men make up just over fourteen
per cent and women, almost eighty-six percent. In management and supervision, men are almost twenty percent and women, eighty percent and among professionals, men are thirteen percent and women twenty-seven percent. So although women form the majority of all groups of job roles, men are relatively over-represented in management and supervisory roles. Furthermore, white workers are significantly over represented amongst managers and supervisors and 'other' workers. Asian workers are significantly over represented amongst professional workers. Black workers form a significantly high proportion of direct care workers followed by a slightly higher proportion of workers from 'other' ethnicities (Hussein 2009). Furthermore, men in non-traditional professions tend to specialize in higher administrative or managerial positions (Williams 1989, 1995) and expect to be promoted (Cree 1996), and also are promoted, more rapidly than their female colleagues (McLean 2003).

The boundaries between paid and unpaid work change over time. For example, some of the caring roles for children which used to be seen as a part of the normal process of parenting have moved into the paid economy with the growth, and professionalization of childcare and the rise of two-earner families. On the other hand, much elder care remains as 'voluntary' activity within the family. Less is known about sexual identity and caring. The literature on informal caring likewise privileges heterosexuality within caring relationships. Despite the gendered nature of care, lesbians caring for their own partners are frequently marginalized and their experience rarely illustrates the caring role (Manthorpe 2003). Lesbians and gay men are thought of as individuals, but not as family members. This reflects the society-wide belief that 'gayness and family are mutually exclusive concepts (Allen and Demon 1995:112, cited by Manthorpe 2003). This is despite the fact that Cronin and King's research (2009) suggests that older gay men are more likely to be carers for parents, partners and friends than heterosexual men.

Within the social care workforce, significant variations are observed in terms of ethnicity, gender and age, highlighting the importance of equality and diversity practices within various social care establishments (Hussein 2009). These illustrate further the gendered processes between the centre and margins of organizational life. These may be literally or metaphorically spatial in the distribution of power and activity between the centre and margins of organizations and management. In summary, what we know about the social care workforce is that front line staff activities are more often staffed by women, central activities more often performed by men leading to the main aim of the organizations tending to be dominantly defined by men (Broadbridge and Hearn 2008, Hussein 2009). The move towards downsizing of public and non-profit social services sector through commissioning and contracting activities plays an important role by providing ongoing support to the private market, getting services ready for privatization, and producing both clients and workers for the for-profit sector (Baines 2004).

Discrimination and sexual harassment

Working from a structural perspective, sexual harassment can be seen as both a gender and a workplace issue which is a practice almost exclusively practised by men directed at women, unsolicited and unreciprocated, frequently involving hierarchical power and is principally about asserting a women's sex role over her function as an employee and the performance of heterosexuality. As such, it seriously restricts women's employment opportunities and undermines their value and status as employees with deleterious economic consequences. Sexual harassment is a key structural mechanism by which men use their power to establish and confirm their dominant economic status over women bringing the value of women's work into question and resulting in a consequent drop in job performance. A number of conduct cases before the General Social Care Council involve inappropriate relationships between service users and social workers and within the work setting (see www.gscc.org.uk). Other research has tended to focus on the risks and outcomes of sexual victimization for a range of service user groups. Further research in this area is warranted in relation to obtaining empirical evidence as well as optimizing research design (Sundaram et al. 2008). The relative silence on the issue of sexual harassment in care services is a reflection of the powerlessness of most women's positions within organizations. It also reflects the lack of personal or economic power to take up the issue and its association with other forms of harassment such as race, sexuality, age and religious belief which often coexist. Many of these themes are echoed in Jeanette Cooperman's chapter in this book (Chapter Six) which documents the institutional abuse of a particular group, that is, women using mental health services. Despite its serious consequences this case has failed to reach the media status of other serious case reviews into organizational failures in care settings.

Sexual harassment and discrimination is an issue which attracts a range of theoretical perspectives and analysis. Some of it reflects the processes in interactions between individuals and individuals' internal mental work (see Joy Trotter, Chapter Eight, in this book for further discussion). Violence is not only direct such as in sexual harassment but also manifests itself in the indirect use of violence through hierarchy and the unfair allocation of resources for example opportunities for training, promotion and other workplace benefits. The intention is not to separate matters such as gender, sexuality and violence, nor privilege these phenomena over other divisions and oppressions within organizations. However, our understandings of relations of oppressions in the social processes of organizations involves an understanding of what happens within them is fundamentally social. These are formed through various social relations, of which gender, sexuality and violation are prime focuses (see Halford and Leonard 2001, Broadbridge and Hearn 2008)

Drawing some conclusions

This chapter has reviewed some of the key discourses in thinking about the relationships between gender, sexuality and organizations within social work and social care. It is a complex landscape which has to be viewed within its historical, social, economic and political context. Whilst wave metaphors are not always useful when talking about political movements that have affected care and its environments, we have moved a long way from a historical era during which feminism and its associated movements had a mass base and influence (Mann and Huffman 2004). Similarly the removal of legal barriers and new public policies within the area of sexuality and sexual identities now offer important opportunities for social work to engage more directly with service users and their networks, so as to ensure the achievement of equality in the assessment and provision of care services (Brown 2008, Cocker and Hafford-Letchfield 2010). Conceptualizing organizational positioning within these critical perspectives can broaden debate about anti-oppressive practice in the over-deterministic framing of services and front line social work. The central question is how current discursive practice in relation to gender and sexuality within the organization might be deconstructed and challenged. The idea that identity is simply a construct of language, discourse, and cultural practices is not sufficient. The goal is to dismantle these fictions and thereby, to undermine hegemonic regimes of discourse.

To affirm identities, as identity politics does, has the potential to merely reproduce and sustain dominant discourses and regulatory power. Some of the features of Foucault's analysis (1984), particularly his focus on subjection, 'othering' and how women might internalize oppressions could be helpful here. New surveillance and control methodologies used in performance management and assessment have taken us away from giving enough attention to achieving equality in social work practice. There are some glimpses of possibilities in developing a more equitable or co-productive relationship with service users (Carr 2007). The move towards personalized services offers opportunities to examine issues of gender and sexuality but also requires an appreciation of the values, connections and desires that bind these social networks together so that there is parallel commissioning and service developments and away from fixed identities (Cant 2009, Cocker and Hafford-Letchfield 2010).

In relation to issues of occupational hierarchy and workforce development, Mavin (2009) suggests that we move away from the metaphor of the glass ceiling towards one of a labyrinth. This is more likely to capture the complex journey that is not a direct passage for women in management and other occupational roles in social work but requires ingenuity, persistence. It requires a very skilled analysis of puzzles and the gendered assumptions that make up the maze of walls and how these change the closer you get to the centre of the labyrinth:

> The labyrinth gives me the opportunity to see different pictures of women's perceived behaviours and women's experiences in management, particularly as they hit the walls of the maze, have to regroup and think, where do I go from here? (Mavin 2009:83).

There are limitations of a modernist approach to resolving some of the issues discussed in this chapter. Millen (1997) argues that through a range of feminist approaches it may be possible to get the best out of both worlds by using post modern insights to continually critique the role of feminist research and the gendered aspects of mainstream research in social work and social care, but using post-modernist ideas to advance feminism's political agenda. Lawlor and Bilson (2010) suggest taking a more relative pluralist approach to enable the incorporation of the voices of both men and women in management and leadership positions, and for those who aspire to such positions to include their interpretations of gender and its influence and importance in social work organizations. I leave you with the words of White (2006:144):

> Only on the basis of thorough analysis will we know whether alternative ways of conceptualizing and organizing services in the interests of women are possible… .[it] would be an analysis of contextualized power relations that would need to be realistic and specific about what is possible in connecting state social work with women's interests.

References

Allen, K. & Demon, D. 1995. The families of lesbian and gay men: A new frontier in family research. *Journal of Marriage and the Family*, 57, 111–27.

Aronson, J. & Smith, K. 2009. Managing restructured social services: expanding the social?, *British Journal of Social Work, Advanced Access*, 40(2), 530–547.

Baines, D. 2004. Caring for nothing: work organization and unwaged labour in social services. *Work, Employment and Society*, 18(2), 267–295.

Bauer, M. & Geront, R.N.M. 1999. The use of humour in addressing the sexuality of elderly nursing home residents. *Sexuality and Disability*, 17(2), 147–155.

Berthoin Antal, A. & Izraeli, D.N. 1993. A global comparison of women in management: women managers in their homelands and as expatriates, in *Women in Management: Trends, Issues, and Challenges in Managerial Diversity*, edited by E. Fagenson. Newbury Park: Sage, 52–96.

Blyth, L. 2005. Not behind closed doors: working in partnership against domestic violence, in *Effective Practice in Health and Social Care: A Partnership Approach,* edited by R. Carnwell & J. Buchanan. Berkshire: The Open University Press.

Broadbridge, A. & Hearn, J. 2008. Gender and management: new directions in research and continuing patterns in practice. *British Journal of Management*. 19(1), S38–S49.

Brown, H.C. 1998 *Social Work and Sexuality: Working with Lesbians and Gay Men*. Basingstoke: Macmillan.

Brown, H.C. 2008. Social work and sexuality, working with lesbians and gay men: what remains the same and what is different? *Practice: Social Work in Action* 20(4), 265–275.

Brown, H.C. & Cocker, C. 2010. *Sexuality in Social Work: Theory and Practice.* London: Sage.

Bryans, P. & Mavin, S. 2003. Women learning to become managers: learning to fit in or to play a different game? *Management Learning*, 34(1), 111–134.

Butler, J. 1990. *Gender Trouble*. London: Routledge.

Cant, B. 2009. Legal outcomes: reflections on the implications of LGBT legal reforms in the UK for health and social care providers. *Diversity in Health and Social Care*, 6(1), 55–62.

Carr, S. 2007. Participation, power, conflict and change: theorizing dynamics of service user participation in the social care system of England and Wales. *Critical Social Policy*, 27(2), 266–276.

Children's Workforce Development Council. 2006. *Options for Excellence: Building the Social Care Workforce of the Future*. Leeds: Children's Workforce Council.

Clarke, J. 2004. *Changing Welfare, Changing States, New Directions in Social Policy.* London: Sage.

Clarke, J. & Newman, J. 1997. *The Managerial State*. London: Sage.

Cocker, C. & Hafford-Letchfield, T. 2000. Critical commentary: out and proud? Social work's relationship with lesbian and gay equality. *British Journal of Social Work*, 40(7), 1996–2005.

Correll, S., Thébaud, S. & Benard, S. 2007. An Introduction to the social psychology of gender. *Advances in Group Processes*, 24, 1–18.

Cree, V.E. 1996. Why do men care?, in *Working with Men: Feminism and Social Work*, edited by K. Cavanagh & V.E. Cree. London: Routledge, 64–86.

Cree, V. 2001. Men and masculinities in social work education, in *Men and Social Work: Theories and Practice*, edited by A. Christie. Basingstoke: Palgrave.

Cronin, A. & King A. 2009. A queer kind of care: some preliminary notes and observations in *LGBT Issues: Looking Beyond Categories*, edited by R.L. Jones & R. Ward. Edinburgh: Dunedin Academic Press.

Department for Children, Schools and Families 2009. *Building a Safe, Confident Future: The Final Report of the Social Work Task Force*. London: Crown Copyright.

Department of Health and Department for Education and Skills 2006. *Options for Excellence*. London: Department of Health Publications.

Department of Health 2000. *No Secrets: Guidance on Developing and Implementing Multi-Agency Policies and Procedures to Protect Vulnerable Adults from Abuse*. London, Department of Health.

Department of Health 2008. *Transforming Social Care: LAC*. London: The Stationary Office.

Department of Health 2008a. *Putting People First: A Shared Vision and Commitment to the Transformation of Adult Social Care*. London: The Stationary Office.

Department of Health 2009 *Shaping the Future of Care Together*. London: Department of Health.

Department of Health. 2009a. *Valuing People Now: A New Three-Year Strategy for People with Learning Disabilities*. London: Department of Health.

Dominelli, L., & McLeod, E. 1989. *Feminist Social Work*. Basingstoke: Macmillan.

Dominelli, L. 2002. *Feminist Social Work Theory and Practice*. London: Palgrave.

Dugmore, P. & Cocker, C. 2008. Legal, social and attitudinal changes: An exploration of lesbian and gay issues in a training programme for social workers in fostering and adoption. *Social Work Education*, 27(1), 159–68.

Eagly, A. & Carli, L. 2007. Women and the labyrinth of leadership. *Harvard Business Review*, 85(9), 62–71.

Equality and Human Rights Commission 2009. *Beyond Tolerance: Making Sexual Orientation a Public Matter*. [Online]. http://www.equalityhumanrights.com/uploaded_files/research/beyond_tolerance.pdf. [Accessed 26 October 2009].

Ferguson, I. 2007. Increasing user choice or privatising risk? The antimonies of personalisation. *British Journal of Social Work*, 37(4), 387–403.

Foster, J. 1999. Women senior managers and conditional power: the case in social services departments. *Women in Management Review*, 14(8), 316–324.

Foucault, M. 1977. *The History of Sexuality: Volume 1 – An Introduction*. London: Penguin.

Foucault, M. 1984 *The History of Sexuality: Volume 3 – The Care of the Self.* London: Penguin.

Gherardi, S. 1994. The gender we think, the gender we do in our everyday organizational lives. *Human Relations*, 47(6), 591–619.

Giddens, A. 1979. *Central Problems in Social Theory*. London: Macmillan.

Gutek, B. 1989. Sexuality in the workplace: key issues in social research and organisational practice, in *The Sexuality of Organisation,* edited by J. Hearn, D. Sheppard, P. Tancred-Sheriff & G. Burrel. London: Sage.

Hafford-Letchfield, T., Chick, N.F., Leonard, K. & Begum, N. 2008. *Leadership and Management in Social Care*. London: Sage.

Hafford-Letchfield, T. 2010. *Social Care Management: Strategy and Business Planning.* London: Jessica Kingsley.

Halford, S. & Leonard, P. 2001. G*ender, Power and Organisations*. Basingstoke: Palgrave.

Hale, J. 1984. Feminism and social work practice, in *The Political Dimensions of Social Work*, edited by N.B. Jordan & N. Parton. Oxford: Basil Blackwell.

Hanmer, J. & Statham, D. 1999. *Women and Social Work: Towards a Woman-Centred Practice.* 2nd edition. Basingstoke: Macmillan.

Harlow, E. 2004. Why don't women want to be social workers any more? New managerialism, post-feminism and the shortage of social workers in social services departments in England and Wales. *European Journal of Social Work*, 7(2), 167–179.

Healy, K. 2002. Managing human services in a market environment; what role for social workers. *British Journal of Social Work*, 32(5), 527–540.

Hearn, J., Sheppard, D., Tancred-Sheriff, P. & Burrell, G. 1989. *The Sexuality of Organisation*. London: Sage.

Hearn, J., & Parkin, W. 2001. *Gender, Sexuality and Violence in Organizations.* London: Sage.

Hicks, S. 2008. Thinking through sexuality. *Journal of Social Work*, 8(1), 65–82.

Her Majesty Government. 2006. *Strong and Prosperous Communities* (Cm 6939–1). Department of Communities and Local Government. London: The Stationary Office.

Hudson, A. 1985. Feminism and social work: resistance or dialogue? *British Journal of Social Work*, 15(6), 635–655.

Hussein, S. 2009. Social care workforce profile: age, gender and ethnicity. Issue 2. *Social Care Workforce Research Unit, Working Paper* (Sept), London: Kings College London.

Jeyasingham, D. 2008. Knowledge/ignorance and the construction of sexuality in social work education. *Social Work Education*, 27(2), 138–51.

Lawler, J. & Bilson, A. 2010. *Social Work Management and Leadership: Managing Complexity with Creativity.* London and New York, NY: Routledge.

Maddock, S. 1999. *Challenging Eomen: Gender, Culture and Organisation.* London: Sage.

Mann, S.A. & Huffman, D.J. 2004. *The impact of post modernism and post structuralism on Third Wave Feminist politics.* Proposed paper for presentation at the American Sociological Association's Annual Meeting in San Francisco, California, August, 2004. http://www.allacademic.com// meta/p_mla_apa_research_citation/1/0/9/9/9/pages109996/p109996-1.php [accessed 30/12/2009].

Manthorpe, J. 2003. Nearest and dearest? The neglect of lesbians in caring relationships. *British Journal of Social Work*, 33(6), 753–768.

Mathieu, C. 2009. Practising gender in organizations: the critical gap between practical and discursive consciousness. *Management Learning*, 40(2), 177–193.

Maynard, M., Afshar, H., Myfawny, F., & Wray, S. 2008. *Women in Later Life: Exploring Race and Ethnicity.* Berkshire: Open University Press.

Martin, P. 2003. 'Said and done' versus 'saying and doing' – gendering practices, practicing gender at work. *Gender and Society*, 17(3), 342–66.

Martin, P. 2006. Practicing gender at work: further thoughts on reflexivity. *Gender, Work and Organization*, 13(3), 254–76.

Mavin, S. 2009 .Navigating the labyrinth: senior women managing emotion. *International Journal of Work Organisation and Emotion*, 3(1), 81–87.

McLean, J. 2003. Men as minority: men employed in statutory social care work. *Journal of Social Work*, 3(1), 45–68.

Miles, N. (not dated) *The Double Glazed Ceiling – Lesbians in the Workplace.* London, Stonewall supported by Lloyds TSB.

Millen, D. 1997. Some Methodological and Epistemological Issues Raised by doing Feminist Research on Non-Feminist Women' Sociological Research Online, *Journal of International Womens Studies*, 2(3). http://www.socreson1ine.org. uk/socresonline/2/3/3.html [Accessed 9/8/2010].

Morrison, T. 2007. Emotional intelligence, emotion and social work: context, characteristics, complications and contribution. *British Journal of Social Work*, 37, 245–263.

Orme, J. 1998. Feminist social work, in *Social work: Themes, Issues and Critical Debates*, edited by R. Adams, L. Dominelli & M. Payne. Basingstoke: Macmillan.

Orme, J. 2009. Feminist Social Work in Social Work Theories and Methods, in *Thinking about Social Work, Theories and Methods for Practice*, edited by M. Gray & S.A. Webb. London: Sage, 65–75.

Scior, K. 2003. Using discourse analysis to study the experiences of women with learning disabilities. *Disability & Society*, 18(6),779–795.

Skills for Care 2008. *The National Minimum Data Set – Social Care (NMDS-SC).* http://www.cwdcouncil.org.uk/nmds-sc [Accessed 1/1/2010].

Stonewall (not dated) Monitoring: how to monitor sexual orientation in the workplace. *Workplace Guides*, www.stonewall.org.uk [Accessed 29/12/09].

Sundaram, V., Laursen, B. & Helweg-Larsen, K. 2008. Is sexual victimization gender specific? The prevalence of forced sexual activity among men and women in Denmark, and self-reported well-being among survivors. *Journal of Interpersonal Violence*, 23(10), 1414–1440.

Weber, M. 1947. *The Theory of Social and Economic Organization*. Translated by A.M. Henderson and Talcott Parsons. London: Collier Macmillan Publishers.

White, V., 2006. *The State of Feminist Social Work*. London: Routledge.

Willams, C.L., 1989. *Gender Differences of Working Women and Men in Non-Traditional Occupations*. California: University of California Press.

Williams, C. 1995. *Still a Man's World: Men Who Do Women's Work*. Berkeley, CA: University of California Press.

Women's National Commission. 2009. *Annual Report, 2008–2009*. London: Women's National Commission.

Yoder, J.D. 2001. Making leadership work more effectively for women. *Journal of Social Issues*, 57(4), 815–28.

Chapter 2

'A Chance to Cut is a Chance to Cure'[1]: Self-harm and Self-protection – A Gay Perspective[2]

Sarah Carr

How do you feel? Alive. Real. Numb. Calm. Satisfied. You smear the blood around. It's sick, but the blood feels real, feels human, feels good. At the same time you feel the pain, you deserve the pain. You tell some people. They say you're manipulative, attention seeking. You believe it. Only serves to make you feel worse. Some people think you're sick, you're weird. One or two may understand, but they're still wary, still shocked by it. Some think you're suicidal. You're not.

Cutting is not attention seeking. It's not manipulation. It's a coping mechanism – a punitive, unpleasant, potentially dangerous one – but it works. It helps me cope with strong emotions that I don't know how to deal with. Don't tell me I'm sick, don't tell me to stop. Don't try to make me feel guilty, that's how I feel already. Listen to me, support me, help me.

'Andrew' in Strong 1998, p. 2.

Introduction

Only a fellow self-harmer like Andrew could articulate so accurately the complex meaning and impact of an act of cutting. When I first read this extract, in a book which brings together case studies and testimonies of self-harm, it was one of few times I had come across somebody describing my own experiences almost exactly. This is why I chose to open this chapter with Andrew's words. I have been self-harming on and off for twenty years, starting with hitting my head in my mid-teens and moving onto cutting when I was eighteen. Since then it has sometimes been the only way to manage acute periods of extreme mental distress. At certain times, no medication, cognitive behavioural training or distraction technique can do what self-cutting can do for me. I may not cut for a long time but I can never say I will not do it again. It is too powerful an intervention and, most importantly,

---

1   The title of a 2001 *Matmos* album (Matador Records), which sampled sounds from surgical procedures.

2   This paper is written in a personal capacity and does not necessarily represent the views of the Social Care Institute for Excellence.

one which I alone control. For me, as it is for many others, self-harm is not about self-destruction, but about self-protection.

In order to try and understand why cutting can be so important for me I have explored some history of medicine, psychological theory and mental health research. In this paper I will share some of my discoveries and several conclusions I have drawn from these explorations relating to my own situation, so that another user/survivor perspective can be added to the growing body of user-generated knowledge on this topic. I acknowledge my perspective is a unique one and I do not claim to speak for all those touched by the same experiences as me, but I hope this chapter will act as a voice crying out from the data. If you are looking for me in the evidence base you will find me here:

- 'Lesbian, gay and bisexual people have been shown to be at greater risk of deliberate self harm' (Department of Health 2007:2)
- 'Lesbian and bisexual women are two times more likely to have deliberately self-harmed' (Department of Health 2007:7)
- 'Our findings show that lesbian, gay and bisexual people are at significantly higher risk of mental disorder, suicidal ideation, substance misuse and deliberate self-harm than heterosexual people' (NIMHE 2007:3)
- In research on female self-harmers, researchers found that 72% did so to control their mind when it is racing and 74% had multiple scars located on their arms (Favazza & Conterio 1989)

Lesbian, gay and bisexual (LGB) people, self-harm and the psychiatric system

> I thought homosexuals were people who were disordered and needed treatment and psychiatric help. And I still do (NHS clinical psychologist [2004 cited in King, Smith and Bartlett 2004:2])

As the data suggest, as someone who is gay, I am a greater risk of developing mental health problems and self-harming than someone who is straight. I also appear to follow one of the patterns common to women who self harm – I generally cut up my arm to control racing thoughts or overwhelming emotions. In order to begin to understand why gay people like me self harm, it is important to recognize that 'discrimination has been shown to be linked to an increase in self-harm in LGB people' (Department of Health 2007:2), rather assuming that our sexual orientation is, in itself, pathological or psychologically abnormal. Our innate inability to conform to the dominant heterosexual culture has led to us attracting the sickness label, as an exploration on the social construction of lesbianism noted: 'Through the diagnosis of mental illness in those who pose a potential threat to the dominant social order, competing conceptualizations of reality are neutralized by assigning them an inferior moral status.... The label of mental illness serves then to invalidate and depoliticize incipient challenges to the dominant version of reality, explaining them in terms of individual weaknesses and personal pathology' (Kitzinger 1995:33). Further to this, sociologists have made the link between social conformity and 'health': 'Conformity – rather than being viewed as a *social* accomplishment – is elevated to the status of "health". Nonconformity is disqualified as "sickness"…' (Pearson 1975:48). This social construction of madness, which relates closely to LGB people's inability to 'play the game', has also been posited by the 'anti-psychiatry' psychiatrist Thomas Szasz, who wrote:

> More precisely, according to the common-sense definition, mental health is the ability to play whatever the game of social living might consist of and play it well. Conversely, to refuse to play or to play badly, means that the person is mentally ill… (Szasz cited in Goffman 1991:317).

Alongside general sociological investigations, specific research into the mental health treatment of LGB people has shown that 'social and political assumptions sometimes lie at the heart of what we regard as mental pathology' (King, Smith & Bartlett 2004:1) and 'the conservative social bias inherent in psychiatry and psychology [has] damaged the lives of gay men and lesbians and provided grounds for discrimination' (King & Bartlett 1999:111). The recent history of psychiatry is littered with examples of LGB people being submitted to appalling treatment supposedly designed to change our sexual orientation, the legacy of which still remains within the mental health system, in psychoanalytic practice and in faith based psychological or group aversion therapies (Bartlett, Smith & King 2009, Carr 2005, Smith, Bartlett & King 2004, King, Smith & Bartlett 2004, Forstein 2004, Bartlett, King & Phillips 2001). In the NHS, damaging experimental physical aversion treatments (such as emetic or electric shock therapy) were still being administered up to the 1970s (King, Smith and Bartlett 2004, Carr 2005), while psychological and psychoanalytical interventions are still being used today by some mental health practitioners in attempts to change a person's sexual orientation: 'A significant minority of mental health professionals are attempting to help lesbian, gay and bisexual clients to become heterosexual. Given the lack of evidence for the efficacy of such treatments, this is likely to be unwise or even harmful' (Bartlett, Smith & King 2009:1). Debates in the UK and US continue about the ethics and efficacy of 'sexual orientation change therapy' by religious groups and therapists working within anti-gay faith-based practice (Forstein 2004). More generally, UK mental health services are operating in a legislative environment which remains unclear about 'conflicting interests between the equality agenda of religious and LGB communities' (COWI 2009), which potentially leaves room for religious groups to provide new forms of aversion therapy – or even revived ancient forms such as exorcism (Tatchell 2009) – to LGB people. However, following a journalistic investigation into conversion therapy (Strudwick 2010) and research which showed that therapists who attempted to change their client's sexual orientation 'paid attention to religious, cultural and moral values causing internal conflict' (Bartlett, Smith & King 2009:1), the British Medical Association declared such therapy discredited and harmful (BMA 2010).

As a key piece of research on the experience of LGB psychiatric patients concluded, 'The definition of same sex attraction as an illness and the development of treatments to eradicate such attraction have had long-term impacts on individuals' (Smith, Bartlett & King 2004:1). This has often lead to LGB people disengaging from or never engaging with mental health services, as we fear the attitudes and treatment we may encounter will harm rather than help us (University of Brighton 2009, Smith, Bartlett & King 2004, Carr 2005, McFarlane 1998): 'Lesbian, gay and bisexual mental health service users are discriminated against and oppressed, not only by the attitudes and behaviour of society at large, but also from within mental health services' (McFarlane 1998:117). Some of us will inevitably conclude that rather than take the risk of entering the potentially homophobic and therefore damaging environment of the psychiatric system, it is safer and more empowering to manage our distress on our own terms. Perhaps that is one of the reasons why LGB people are more likely to develop methods like self-harm to manage periods of distress or self-medicate through drug and alcohol use. The potential effects of an oppressive psychiatric system for LGB people who self-harm are echoed in the words of Louise Pembroke, a survivor activist and founder of the National Self-Harm Network, who makes the explicit link between self-harm and powerlessness, particularly in relation to being in the mental health system:

> As an in-patient, as an out-patient … I was continuously harming myself… I started self-harming because I felt powerless. It was a reaction to the treatment I was receiving. I would cut myself up as a way of expressing my pain and anger. Also out of sheer frustration, as a way of dealing with all the things that went on … (Pembroke, 1996:170).

Self-harm and the 'spoiled identity'

The Department of Health has clearly recognized the impact of discrimination on the mental health of LGB people (Department of Health 2007), and yet the mental health system is one of the sites for some of the most damaging forms of discrimination. Given this, some lesbian gay and bisexual people construct different ways to look after ourselves, and even if our actions and 'behaviour' further marginalize us, they are about our personal choice and control. Self-harm is often about responding to powerlessness and distress. As one author remarked, 'given the extremely negative attitudes held by the public and by mental health professionals, it is remarkable that lesbians and gay men have adjusted so well' (Rothblum 1994:214) – that is, given our situation and experiences it is surprising that not more of us are mad.

It is difficult to explain to people who have not grown up gay, conscious of an innate sense of difference as a child and then aware of predominant same-sex attraction in early adolescence, how such experiences can profoundly impact on the early development of your psychology and identity in a society which requires conformity and in a culture in which heterosexuality is the dominant defining force.

The lesbian feminist Adrienne Rich described the consequences of 'compulsory heterosexuality' for some women and asserted that 'lesbian existence comprises both the breaking of a taboo and the rejection of a compulsory way of life', albeit it 'lived without access to any knowledge of a tradition, a continuity, a social underpinning' (Rich 1980 cited in Humm 1992:178). Having no familial or ancestral history, an immediately accessible 'community' or many visible positive role models to strengthen our sense of self or to empower us in the face of social discrimination and isolation continues to have a profound negative impact on LGB people of all ages. In a paper arguing the importance of parental support for LGB people, two US mental health practitioners with a gay son, alerted fellow practitioners to the following defining issue for lesbian and gay people:

> As minorities, they are also somewhat unique in that they represent a marginalized segment of our society, whose parents do not share their minority status. Consequently, they are confronted with the additional challenge of not only being stigmatized by society at large but also the prospect of being outcast in their own homes (Goldfried & Goldfried 2001:684).

Additionally, homophobic bullying in schools, which is now recognized as a widespread and serious issue (DCSF 2007), means that young LGB people often have to operate in a environments of fear and potential violence, largely unprotected by teachers (Stonewall 2007, Stonewall 2009). Research on the social-developmental factors affecting young LGB people indicates that exposure to such conditions may cause long-term damage to our mental health and psychological development because:

> At a time when other adolescents are discovering how to express themselves socially, those youth who identify as lesbian or gay, but wish to remain hidden, are learning to conceal large parts of themselves from their family and friends (Rivers & Carragher 2003:382).

In the 1980s when I was discovering I was gay, I was also discovering what society thought of me and learning about my assigned inferior moral status. The Conservative government under Margaret Thatcher was waging a political and moral war against the likes of me, resulting in Section 28 of the 1988 Local Government Act. This Act made it unlawful for local authorities to: 'a) intentionally promote homosexuality or publish material with the intention of promoting homosexuality, b) promote teaching in any maintained school of the acceptability of homosexuality as a pretended family relationship' (Warwick et al. 2001). In the media I read that I was perverted, ugly, mentally ill, sick, morally corrupt, murderous, a threat to the family, children and to the social order. At church I learned that I was 'intrinsically disordered' (Pope Paul VI 1975), against nature, condemned by God, suffering from 'an intrinsic moral evil' (Ratzinger 1986) and in danger of committing 'sin crying to heaven for vengeance' (Catholic Church 2002). At school I learned that non-conformity attracted the 'lesbian' label which singled you out for marginalization and bullying by both genders alike. In my family I realized that I would be rejected for who I really was and that my parents would never endorse or celebrate my relationships. In short, as one friend put it, 'when we were growing up we experienced a violation of our sexual identity' and we became alienated and withdrawn, with diminishing self-worth, power and hope. As a consequence some of us developed mental health problems and it may even be true to say that some of us experienced significant trauma as gay children and young people. When I reflect on my formative experiences as a gay woman, my struggle with mental distress and self-worth starts to make sense: 'Our experiences do not merely link us to the outside world; they are us and they are the world for us; they make us part of the world ….' (Bronowski 1971, quoted in Kaufman 1993:3).

LGB people were and, despite the legislative and social progress that has been made in the past decade (EHRC 2009), are still what Erving Goffman refers to as a 'shamed group' whose experiences can result in the development of a 'spoiled identity' which requires us to engage in 'stigma management' to protect ourselves and operate in society (Goffman 1990). Some have been impressed by the 'ability of lesbians and gay men to cope adaptively with stigma' (Rothblum, 1994:214) but enforced adaptation has too often compromised our lives, mental health, identity and sense of self. Goffman's theories about the management of a spoiled identity have helped me understand my situation, as have the theories on the psychology of shame (Kaufman 1993). The internalization of shame, invisibility and the risks of being visible have long been psychological and ontological issues for LGB people. Most acutely, shame and fear can affect the ability of LGB people to be open with people closest to us and relationships which should ensure mental wellbeing become a cause for chronic anxiety, as Goffman notes: 'the individual's intimates can become just the persons from whom he [sic] is most concerned with concealing something shameful; the situation of the homosexual [sic] provides an illustration… '(Goffman 1990:71). As Goldfried and Goldfried argue 'It is important to note that one's sexual orientation, per se, does not contribute to suicidality, but rather the depression and hopelessness resulting from the rejection by others does' (Goldfried and Goldfried 2001:683). Self-harmers have been very clear why we do what we do: 'Powerlessness, worthlessness, helplessness and control are the underlying factors. The issue of self-worth is critical. There is a collapse of self-worth and that is when self-harm occurs' (Pembroke cited in Laurance 2003:152). For those LGB people who have critically low self-worth and scant support, self-harm would seem an inevitable way of dealing with mental distress.

Reclaiming cutting, blood and the self

The powerlessness that has often been experienced by many LGB people like me is not to do with having power over others but rather it is the 'need to feel in command of one's life' (Kaufman 1993:83). For LGB people who have not felt in command of their lives for all the reasons discussed here, self-harm can be a liberating way to deal with the mental distress arising from our situation. It is an intervention which is in your command alone; it is an entirely autonomous act with instantaneous effects. Cutting can make you become visible to yourself and seeing your own blood can be extremely cathartic if you've been conditioned to hide your emotions as shameful: 'I would cut myself instead of crying. Because when the blood ran away, it felt like tears. The injury was doing the crying for me' (Pembroke 1996:170). Self-harm is recognized as a mechanism to control distress and regulate emotion, but harmers like me may also say that cutting makes them feel more 'real', which in clinical terms is often seen as a response to dissociation (that is feeling disconnected from reality) (Tolmunen et al. 2008, Brodsky, Cloitre & Dulit 1995). It could be argued that LGB people like myself, who, as young people were excluded from every almost form of social and cultural validation and afraid of the consequences of revealing their sexual orientation to close friends and family, had to detach from reality to cope. As a result, in later life we can develop and endure dissociative states, and many of us have been suicidal (myself included) at some point in our lives (Johnson et al. 2007).

The pervasive silencing and invisibility of our lives can result in some of us actually feeling unreal or invisible – I know this has been the case for me. Seeing something as corporeal as my own blood and scarred skin helps alleviate my sense of invisibility; having sole agency over the cutting, bloodletting and scarring allows me to feel alive and in control. Through the action and consequence of cutting I become real and visible to myself, if no one else: 'Deliberate self-harm as a means of validating the self… for many individuals who have been traumatized… [for whom] there was no recognition of their experiences and the events that damaged them may have been actively denied' (Swales 2004). This sense of silencing is powerfully reflected in the stark inscription on a memorial in Berlin to the gay people who were persecuted and murdered by the Nazis: 'Totgeschlagen – Totgeschwiegen (*Struck Dead – Hushed Up*)'. Scarring too can be important because it is both a visible symbol of hidden distress and a mark of healing, and by the same token it is probably no coincidence that body piercing and tattooing are an important part of certain lesbian and gay subcultures:

> Self-mutilation may also be therapeutic because of the symbolism associated with the formation of scar-tissue, scar tissue indicates that healing has occurred….
> The cutter in effect performs a primitive sort of self-surgery complete with tangible evidence of healing… Just as a significant event symbolically can be burned in one's memory, so too it literally can be burned into one's skin (Favazza 1996:280).

Self-cutting and bloodletting, then, can be 'a life-sustaining and sanity-maintaining way of managing inner states' (Strong 1998:44) and individuals like me who do it for this reason often begin self-harming independently and without knowledge of other harmers' practice. But far from being the abnormal, deviant and taboo behaviour that many clinicians see it as (see for example Patel, Benaknin & Tsao 2006), self-harm 'seems to tap into deeply embedded sentiments of healing, religion and interpersonal amity' (Favazza in Strong 1998:xi). Blood customs and healing are ancient human responses to sickness and distress (Favazza 1996) and blood is one of the 'four humours', the theory upon which pre-modern understanding of the body and medicine was based. In ancient Greek medicine bloodletting or 'phlebotomy' was seen as a panacea for both physical and mental illness. The classical philosopher and physician 'Galen… judged phlebotomy an essential remedy called for in any severe disease' (Kuriyama 1995:11). While bloodletting as an intervention for physical conditions was declining in Western medicine during the nineteenth century, its practice continued in psychiatry, as the medical historian Roy Porter noted, 'in the New World, Benjamin Rush of Philadelphia, the physician officially acknowledged by the American Psychiatric association as "the father of American psychiatry", held that practically all mental disorders were due to vitiated blood. His systematic remedy was bloodletting' (Porter 2002:127). In an 1854 volume entitled 'An Examination of the Practice of Bloodletting in Mental Disorders', Pliny Earle surveyed the contemporary psychiatric practice, observing that:

> The effect of local bleeding is more favourable [than the general bleeding as recommended by Benjamin Rush] and may sometimes procure relief from distressing symptoms and afford an abatement of excitement…Local bleeding is usually prescribed to procure present relief, rather than with the expectation of permanent benefit (Earle 1854:13–14).

Blood and bleeding were therefore once central to psychiatric practice and implements such as scarificators, cups, lancets and 'mechanical leeches' remain on display at the Museum of the Royal College of Surgeons or the Wellcome Collection in London. It is an irony then that those of us who self-harm in order to manage our mental states are seen as an aberration or personality disordered by the very system that once used phlebotomy as a form of treatment. One psychiatrist has hypothesized that 'bulimic purging fills the psychological niche occupied for so many centuries by therapeutic bloodletting' (Cosman 1986:1189) and I would argue that therapeutic bloodletting has also been reclaimed more directly by self-cutters, many of whom identify themselves as lesbian, gay or bisexual.

Supporting LGB people who self-harm: the challenge of personalisation

> In the fight to be free to be who you really are … what you're seeking is, like, a lovely life (Mental health service user in MIND 2009:11).

As a gay woman with mental health problems who self-harms, I do not and cannot 'play the game' or be cured according to the traditional medical model. I do, however, know what helps and what harms me, yet rarely has my personal expertise and insight been sought and used by mental health practitioners. As with countless other individuals in my situation, my case is too complex for restrictive diagnostic labels and I may not respond well to pre-determined, imposed therapeutic regimes (such as cognitive or dialectical behavioural therapy), where I have no choice or control. Armando Favazza, in his seminal book exploring self-harm and body modification in religion, culture and psychiatry emphasized the need to understand the complicated nature of self-harm:

> Self-mutilation is a multi-determined behaviour and can be understood only by attention to interactions among psychological and biological functioning, the environment and social setting, and the overarching web of culture (Favazza 1996:282).

In other words, simplistic approaches like giving us stigmatizing diagnoses, telling us to stop it and judging us as moral deficients who should not have a voice will not help us. My personal plea to mental health practitioners would be to treat us as individuals with unique histories and experiences who have different ways of managing our mental states. As one of those different ways of managing distress, self-harm needs to be understood as a complex response to those histories and experiences. Actions like cutting and bloodletting are part of a long tradition, which when carried out by psychiatrists one hundred and fifty years ago were accepted as part of standard practice rather than seen as extreme or abnormal.

The Department of Health has recognized that although LGB people are at higher risk of mental health problems and self-harm, mental health services are not yet supportive, affirming environments for us: 'An awareness of the mental health needs of LGB people should become a standard part of training for health and social work professionals' (NIMHE 2007:3). This training should be co-produced with LGB people with direct experience of mental distress and self-harm, particularly in the context of the personalization agenda which aims to: put people and their chosen outcomes rather than processes and systems first; to make health and social care services more responsive to the needs of people who use them; and to promote the recognition of the expertise of people using services so they can co-design and co-produce the care and support that is right for them (HM Government 2007; Carr 2008; DH 2010). Specific mental health policy proposals as outlined in 'New Horizons' (HM Government 2009) focus on the need to tackle stigma and to promote personalized care and innovation. Mental health services, along with health and social care in general, therefore need to be far more responsive to, understanding and respectful of LGB people, be they people using or working in services (Hunt, Cowan & Chamberlain 2007, Fish 2006). This includes working with us to understand and manage our mental health distress, which will mean being open to innovative ways of working that some practitioners may perceive as 'risky'.

Mental health service users and survivors have been very clear that 'their support services should not rely on a passive illness model. When they need support, they do not want at the same time to lose their sense of a positive identity' (MIND 2009:11). Achieving and maintaining a positive identity and protective self-worth is vital for the wellbeing of LGB people who have mental health problems, especially self harmers. This requires empowering, person-centred working built on long-term, trusting and mutually respectful relationships with mental health practitioners and social care workers. The mental health system still mirrors and compounds the isolation and discrimination experienced by LGB people in wider society and 'there is a need for… front line health professionals… to challenge discriminatory practices that pathologizes LGBT people' (Johnson et al. 2007:6). Similarly, institutionalized discriminatory practices also impact on people who self-harm where people are told to stop rather than supported to minimize harm and be enabled to 'self-injure in a safer, more controlled way' (Spandler & Warner 2007:30). LGB people who self harm could benefit from being able to choose appropriate support workers or personal assistants and use advance directives or agreements to maintain control over what happens when they self-harm (Spandler & Vick 2006). The 'personalization' reforms in health and social care mean that policy makers and practitioners need to reconceptualize their role as enabling greater capacity for choice, control and independent living for *all* those who use or may need to use mental health, care and support services. The challenge is to work sensitively and creatively with individuals who have been among the most judged, marginalized, silenced and stigmatized while resisting and challenging the institutional drive towards 'efficient and effective management of "deviant" populations which seek to integrate [people] … into political, economic and ideological structures over which they ultimately have little control' (Spandler 2007:25).

References

Bartlett, A., King, M. & Phillips, P. 2001. Straight talking: an investigation of the attitudes and practice of psychoanalysts and psychotherapists in relation to gays and lesbians. *British Journal of Psychiatry*, 179, 545–49.

Bartlett, A., Smith, G. & King, M. 2009. The response of mental health professionals to clients seeking help to change or redirect same-sex sexual orientation. *BMC Psychiatry*, 9, 11.

British Medical Association 2010. In: S. Cassidy. BMA declares that 'conversion therapy' for gays is harmful. *The Independent*, Friday 2 July [online]. Available at: http://www.independent.co.uk/life-style/health-and-families/health-news/bma-declares-that-conversion-therapy-forgays-is-harmful-2016391.html (accessed November 2010).

Brodsky, B., Cloitre, M. & Dulit, R. 1995. Relationship of dissociation to self-mutilation and childhood abuse in borderline personality disorder. *American Journal of Psychiatry*, 152, 1788–92.

Carr, S. 2005. 'The sickness label infected everything we said': lesbian and gay perspectives on mental distress, in *Social Perspectives in Mental Health*, edited by J. Tew. London: Jessica Kingsley, 168–183.

Carr, S. 2008. *Personalisation: a rough guide*. London: SCIE.

Catholic Church 2002. *Catechism of the Catholic Church*. London/New York: Burns & Oates.

Cosman, B. 1986. Bloodletting as purging behaviour. *American Journal of Psychiatry*, 143(9), 1188–89.

COWI 2009. *The social situation concerning homophobia and discrimination on grounds of sexual orientation in the United Kingdom*. Copenhagen: Danish Institute for Human Rights.

DCSF 2007. *Homophobic bullying: Safe to Learn: Embedding anti-bullying work in schools*. London: Department for Children Schools and Families.

Department of Health 2007. *Briefing 9: Mental health issues within lesbian, gay and bisexual (LGB) communities*. London: Department of Health.

Department of Health 2010. A vision for adult social care: capable communities and active citizens London: Department of Health.

Earle, P. 1854. *An Examination of the Practice of Bloodletting in Mental Disorders*. New York: Samuel S. & William Wood.

EHRC 2009. *Beyond Tolerance: Making sexual orientation a public matter*. London: Equalities and Human Rights Commission.

Favazza, A. & Conterio, K. 1989. Female habitual self-mutilators. *Acta Scandinavica*, 79, 283–89.

Favazza, A. 1996. *Bodies Under Siege: Self-mutilation and Body Modification in Culture and Psychiatry*. Baltimore: The Johns Hopkins University Press.

Fish, J. 2006. *Heterosexism in Health and Social Care*. Basingstoke: Palgrave Macmillan.

Forstein, M. 2004. Pseudoscience of sexual orientation change therapy. *British Medical Journal (Clinical Research Ed)*, 328, E287.

Goffman, E. 1991. *Asylums*. London: Penguin.

Goffman, E. 1990. *Stigma: Notes on the Management of Spoiled Identity*. London: Penguin.

Goldfried, M. & Goldfried, A. 2001. The importance of parental support in the lives of gay, lesbian and bisexual individuals. *Psychotherapy in Practice*, 57(5), 681–93.

HM Government 2007. *Putting People First: A Shared Vision and Commitment to the Transformation of Adult Social Care*. London: HM Government.

HM Government 2009. *New Horizons: A Shared Vision for Mental Health*. London: Department of Health.

Humm, M. 1992. *Feminisms: A Reader*. Edited by M. Humm. London: Harvester Wheatsheaf.

Hunt, R. Cowan, K. & Chamberlain, B. 2007. *Being the Gay One: Experiences of Lesbian, Gay and Bisexual People Working in the Health and Social Care Sector*. London: Stonewall.

Johnson, K., Faulkner, P., Jones, H. & Welsh, E. 2007. *Understanding Suicide and Promoting Survival in LGBT Communities* Brighton: University of Brighton/MindOut.

Kaufman, G. 1993. *The Psychology of Shame: Theory and Treatment of Shame Based Syndromes*. London: Routledge.

King, M. & Bartlett, A. 1999. British psychiatry and homosexuality. *British Journal of Psychiatry*, 175, 106–13.

King, M. & McKeown, E. 2003. *Mental Health and Social Wellbeing of Gay Men, Lesbians and Bisexuals in England and Wales: A Summary of Findings*. London: MIND.

King, M., Smith, G. & Bartlett, A. 2004. Treatments of homosexuality in Britain since the 1950s – an oral history: the experience of professionals. *British Medical Journal*, 328, 429.

Kitzinger, C. 1995. *The Social Construction of Lesbianism*. London: Sage.

Kuriyama, S. 1995. Interpreting the history of bloodletting. *Journal of the History of Medicine and Allied Sciences*, 50(1), 11–46.

Laurance, J. 2003. *Pure Madness: How Fear Drives the Mental Health System*. London: Routledge.

McFarlane, L. 1998. *Diagnosis Homophobic: The Experiences of Lesbians, Gay Men and Bisexuals in Mental Health Services*. London: PACE.

MIND 2009. *Personalisation in Mental Health: Creating a Vision – Views of Personalisation from People who use Mental Health Services*. London: MIND.

NIMHE 2007. *Mental Disorders, Suicide and Deliberate Self-Harm in Lesbian, Gay and Bisexual people*. London: NIMHE.

Patel, S., Benaknin, J. & Tsao, C. 2006. Ritualistic excoriation and blood-letting resulting in anemia in borderline personality disorder. *General Hospital Psychiatry*, 28(6), 539–540.

Pearson, G. 1975. *The Deviant Imagination: Psychiatry, Social Work and Social Change*. London: Macmillan

Pembroke, L. 1996. It helped that someone believed me, in *Speaking Our Minds: An Anthology*, edited by J. Read & J. Reynolds. London: Macmillan, 168–173.

Pope Paul VI 1975. *Persona Humana: Declaration on Certain Questions Concerning Sexual Ethics*. Vatican City: Sacred Congregation for the Doctrine of the Faith.

Porter, R. 2002. *Madness: A Brief History*. Oxford: OUP

Ratzinger, J. 1986. *Letter to the Bishops of the Catholic Church on the Pastoral Care of Homosexual Persons*. Vatican City: Sacred Congregation for the Doctrine of the Faith.

Rivers, I. & Carragher, D. 2003. Social-developmental factors affecting lesbians and gay youth: a review of cross-national research findings. *Children and Society*, 17, 374–385.

Rothblum, E. 1994. 'I only read about myself on bathroom walls': The need for research on the mental health of lesbians and gay men. *Journal Consulting and Clinical Psychology*, 62(2), 213–220.

Smith, G., Bartlett, A. & King, M. 2004. Treatments of homosexuality in Britain since the 1950s – an oral history: the experience of patients. *British Medical Journal*, 328,427.

Spandler, H. & Vick, N. 2006 Opportunities for independent living using direct payments in mental health. *Health and Social Care in the Community*, 14(2), 107–115.

Spandler, H. & Warner, S. 2007. *Beyond Fear and Control*. Ross-on-Wye: PCCS Books.

Spandler, H. 2007. Individualised funding, social inclusion and the politics of mental health. *Journal of Critical Psychological Counselling*, 7(1), 18–27.

Stonewall 2007. *The School Report: the experience of young gay people in Britain's schools*. London: Stonewall.

Stonewall 2009. *Teachers' Report: homophobic bullying in Britain's schools*. London: Stonewall.

Strong, M. 1998. *A Bright Red Scream: Self-Mutilation and the Language of Pain* London: Virago.

Strudwick, P. 2010. The ex-gay files: the bizarre world of gay-to-straight conversion. *The Independent*, 1 February [online]. Available at: http://www.independent.co.uk/life-style/health-and-families/features/the-exgay-files-the-bizarre-world-of-gaytostraight-conversion-1884947. html (accessed November 2010.)

Swales, M. 2004. *Pain and Deliberate Self-Harm* [online: Wellcome Trust]. Available at: http://www.wellcome.ac.uk/en/pain/microsite/culture4.html [accessed 6 January 2010].

Tatchell, P. 2009. *Exorcism of gays in the UK: Protest Against Abuse by Fundamentalist Christians*. [online]. http://www.petertatchell.net/religion/Exorcism%20of%20gays%20in%20the%20UK.htm [accessed 6 January 2010].

Tolmunen, T., Rissanen, M.L., Hintikka, J. et al. 2008. Dissociation, self-cutting and other self-harm behaviour in a general population of Finnish adolescents. *Journal of Nervous and Mental Disorders*, 196(10), 768–771.

University of Brighton 2009. *Count Me In Too Community Summary: Mental Health and LGBT Lives*. Brighton: Count Me In Too LGBT Research Information Desk.

Warwick, I., Aggerton, P. & Douglas, N. 2001. Playing it safe: addressing the emotional and physical health of lesbian and gay pupils in the UK. *Journal of Adolescence*, 24(1), 129–140.

Chapter 3

Researching Sexuality and Ageing

Rhiannon Jones

Introduction

For the past thirty years, initially as a practitioner and then as an academic within the field of social work, I have been committed to working with, and raising the profile of, issues concerning older age. My journey has highlighted for me the fact that certain issues in relation to older people are either poorly understood or ignored. I feel that this is particularly true in respect of sexuality, a view which has in turn acted as a catalyst and focus for my PhD research study. The research study is in two parts, with the aim of the first part being to identify any methodological issues in researching sexuality and ageing. This is in direct response to the dearth of literature within this area as well as informing the methodology of the second part of the research study, whose broad aim is to explore older women's experiences of their sexuality and the impact it may have had on their sense of self. This chapter focuses on the findings of the first part of the study and uses the recommendations to reflect on how they can inform social work practice.

Engaging in research with older people around the issues of sexuality raises general concerns ranging from the belief that the sensitivity of the topic makes the research methodologically too difficult (Pointon 1997, Gott 2001, Gott and Hinchliff 2003), through to a perception that sexuality is incompatible with and antithetical to older age (Gott 2005). These views are supported by particular perceptions of older people's sexuality which, within western society, are constructed by two dominant discourses, that of 'asexuality' and 'the sexy oldie'. The assumption of asexuality is created and maintained by a range of different structural and cultural aspects of western society and is reflected in the continuing exclusion of older people's sexuality from some major areas of policy and sexuality research (Minichiello et al. 2004, Delamater and Sill 2005, Gott 2006, Bywater and Jones 2007, Hinchliff 2009). Many research studies involving older people do not address issues of sexuality and vice versa (Gott and Hinchliff 2003). Although themes of silence and invisibility have tended to dominate sexuality in later life (Bywater and Jones 2007), there has over the years been a growing body of research giving recognition to older people's sexuality. The focus of this recognition however has been the quantifying of (hetero)sexual activity in terms of *'which older people do it and how often?'* (Gott 2005:55) and viewing issues of sexuality through a narrow medicalized lens. This perspective has gained stature fuelled by the belief that sexual activity in later life not only is a statement of successful and healthy ageing (Katz and Marshall 2004) but also a way of defying older age and in effect, *'choosing not to be old'* (Biggs 1997:553). It is argued that these factors together with the promotion and consumption of erectile dysfunction drugs such as Viagra have created the *'sexy oldie'* (Gott 2005:23).

The two discourses are not however competing, but interrelated in that older people who cannot adhere to a youthfully defined and problem free sexual image of the 'sexy oldie' forfeit the right to a sexuality by being perceived or rendered asexual. People whose sexuality intersects with a perceived 'old' age through illness, disability and mental frailty have their (hetero)sexuality delegitimized and are deemed unfit to be sexual citizens. Older women's experiences of sexuality particularly struggle to be recognized within the preceding context. The concept of the 'sexy oldie' is driven by the emphasis on erectile dysfunction and the ability of the man to perform (hetero)sexually (Loe 2004). Older women fight invisibility on all fronts in terms of sexuality and ageing. For older women the 'sexy oldie' cannot be viewed or experienced as 'disrupting' the asexual discourse. Older women's sexuality, sexual desire and activity continue to be at best marginalized and at worst invisible. Both discourses serve as an oppressive context for any research study wanting to enable older women to narrate their experiences of their sexuality within the context of their own ageing.

Researching sexuality in older age: what is already known?

In order to raise the profile of older women's sexuality through accessing narratives and developing theories that are credible and meaningful to an increasingly growing and diverse population, there is urgent need for a debate around some of the methodological issues of researching sexuality in older age. The context of older people's sexuality referred to in the introduction of this chapter seems to have resulted in a lack of literature focusing on the issues and challenges raised by researching sexuality and ageing with only a few researchers exploring the issues in any depth. Jones (2005) considers a range of methodological issues with particular focus on recruitment of older people and the impact of the sensitivity of the topic of sexuality. Pugh and Jones (2007) consider some of the difficulties of researching sexuality with older lesbians and gay men in relation to recruitment, representative sampling and different methods of data collection. Lee (2008) considers the impact of the researcher on the interview process when undertaking research with older gay men and also highlights the general 'lack of reflection on the research process' (para 1.5) within research studies in the field of sexuality and ageing. Other writers in the field of sexuality research are not plentiful and tend to focus on younger people (e.g. Hutchinson et al. 2002), covering a range of issues including, the researcher's impact on the research process and vice versa (Israel 2002, Perry et al. 2004, Poole et al. 2004, La Pastina 2006), researching non-heterosexual relationships (Heaphy et al. 1998), collaborative research (Wahab

2003), ethical dilemmas and recruitment (Ringheim 1995, Sanders 2006), and data collection (Fish 1999, Frith 2000, Harding and Peel 2007).

Researching sexuality and ageing: what is there to discover?

With a limited amount of literature discussing the issues and challenges of researching sexuality and ageing, it was important to undertake a qualitative study with an aim to discover how to develop good research practice and ensure the success of research in this area. Initially a purposive sample of 14 participants was recruited to take part in individual semi-structured interviews. The participants were made up of six older women over 70 years of age and eight researchers who were working within the field of sexuality research. The interview schedule was based on seven key aspects of the research process, which included level of importance, gaps in knowledge, influence of society's views of sexuality and ageing, language of sexuality, recruitment of participants, data collection methods, and the researcher's influence on the research process. They had been identified through an extensive review of literature within the field of researching sexuality and ageing and reflected the different stages of the research process with the exclusion of data analysis, writing-up and dissemination of findings (McLeod 2003). These aspects constituted the coding framework under which themes were developed in relation to researching sexuality and ageing using a thematic analysis (Braun and Clarke 2006).

A crucial element to this research study was the inclusion of older women as research participants in recognition that they continue to struggle to be included in sexuality research on any level and in particular to be included in influencing the methodology of future research. The participation of older women as 'advisors on methodology' (Peace 1999:2) reflected a commitment to participative research at a consultation level (Hanley et al. 2004). The older women participants were regarded as 'knowledgeable experts' on the experiences of their own ageing and sexuality, which would help to produce research findings that were relevant and important to older women participants in future research. Also the women's participation in this research study challenged the stereotypical perceptions of sexuality and ageing being unable to co-exist by highlighting older women's interest in discussing sexuality and how the topic could be researched successfully.

It was felt that both researcher and older women participants usefully offered different perspectives in the form of providers and users of research respectively, and that these differing perspectives represented pieces of the same picture giving an additional richness to the data. Therefore the data from all participants was analysed as a whole as opposed to being presented as a comparative study of the views of researchers and older women. For the purposes of this chapter, however, emphasis will be placed on the older women whose voices, through the use of quotations, will be used to support the themes. It is worth pointing out that during the analysis it became apparent that the research processes' 'macro' aspects of importance, gaps, sexuality, ageing and society, and language, were an influential context to the 'micro' aspects of recruitment, data collection and researcher influence. The remainder of the chapter will present a summary of the findings of the study, and although each aspect is presented separately in order to aid the structure of the discussion, their interrelatedness is assumed and where possible highlighted. The themes identified in the analysis are highlighted in single inverted commas. Recommendations are also offered for research practice in this area which could also be applied to social work practice when engaging older women in conversations about their experiences of their sexuality.

Sexuality and ageing research: Why is it important?

All participants felt that researching sexuality should be an important part of the ageing and later life research agenda. There was a recognition that older women's sexuality struggled to 'establish a presence', in both social and research worlds. The older women participants spoke of a lack of discussion and a silence around sexuality within their own social networks, whilst the researcher participants identified older people's sexuality as a neglected and under-researched area. Research focusing on sexuality and ageing was considered by the participants to have an important role in challenging this lack of presence through 'breaking the silence' and 'bringing discussion out into the open' in relation to sexuality. Research enables older women in particular to be taken seriously in terms of voicing and expressing their sexuality.

> I do think that the research should be done and published and talked about. I do feel that the images of older women and sexuality are incredibly important…. I mean older women and their sexuality should be open much more to expression (Older woman, 71).

A number of the participants felt that it was important for research not only to 'establish a presence' in terms of sexuality, but also to establish a certain type of presence which challenges myths, images and information that do not adequately reflect the experiences of older women. Another important part therefore of the role of research in sexuality and ageing is 'making a difference' which involves challenging perceptions, changing attitudes and creating a better understanding across generations towards older women and their experiences of their own sexuality. It could be suggested that researching sexuality and ageing addresses the concept of 'catalytic validity' (Lather 1991:68), with its potential to empower older women as well as stimulate and promote change.

> I think it {researching sexuality and ageing} would be good because it would expose some of the myths and might enable more discussion, more acknowledgement that it {being sexual}is perfectly normal whereas at the

moment I think people like me feel abnormal. I certainly feel I've been made to feel abnormal because I'm not like what the media puts across to us (Older Woman, 72).

Sexuality and ageing: Where are the knowledge gaps?

The majority of the researcher participants felt that the knowledge gap in relation to researching sexuality and ageing was in the 'type of research' with quantitative methods dominating the field. It was felt that more qualitative research studies were needed to encourage older women to talk about their experiences of their sexuality. DeLamater and Sill (2005:24) support this view, arguing that 'qualitative research methods need to be used to complement quantitative methods in order to learn how older people think about sexuality'. The findings also drew attention to the fact that the voice of the medic, health professional and sexologist also dominates research studies making it difficult to access the diversity of experiences and meanings that sexuality has in later life.

Contrasting with this the older women participants had very specific but wide ranging questions about sexuality that they wanted future research to explore, including for example, how older women cope with a loss of a sexual partner, how older women feel about their bodies, what sexual practices older women engage in, and how personal histories and societal pressures affect older women's sexuality. A common focus of interest across these areas of enquiry involved the concept of change where there was an assumption by participants that changes in sexuality did take place during the ageing process. There was also a sense from the participants that they felt it was important for research to explore not only what the changes may be but also where the changes may lead older women.

> How the definition {of sexuality}, whatever definition they give, is different from what they said about themselves 30 years ago… well what they {older women} mean by sexuality and what does it mean for them in this stage of their life and do they think it's still important… to get them to talk about what sexuality and sensuality means to them (Older Woman, 78).

The key theme 'transitions in sexuality' pulls the areas of enquiry together as well as reflecting a sense that the changes involve movement that may lead to growth, development and possible transformation of sexuality within the context of ageing, in terms of its form, shape and appearance. Deacon et al. (1995:507) state that it is important to view sexuality as being constructed over a lifetime and research studies that support this concept 'may provide knowledge that challenges the tendency to conceptualize sexuality and aging as continual combatants'.

The research process: How does society's views of sexuality and ageing impact?

Most of the participants recognized that researching sexuality takes place within a context which is made up of dominant ideas and images of sexuality and ageing which can impact negatively on the research process. The researcher participants for example experienced a 'lack of support' for their research, particularly qualitative research, ranging from difficulty in acquiring mainstream funding to doubt being raised by their colleagues and peers of the importance and usefulness of such research. Okami (2002) highlights the lack of financial and professional support experienced by sexuality researchers, stating that the latter often experience working within a hostile academic environment where they have difficulties in, gaining funding, having their work accepted by the better journals, and securing promotion. Israel (2002) argues that researchers need to employ strategies to survive the stigma of sexuality research, such as by forming a support network with other sexuality researchers which may in turn help to secure future careers.

The older women participants gave examples of 'negative attitudes' they had experienced towards their own sexuality, such as sexuality being predominantly associated only with younger people, older women being portrayed as asexual and the lack of information about sexual matters for older people. There was the view that negative attitudes may have an unhelpful impact on older people expressing their sexuality.

> I don't think anything to do with people should be off-limits and I am interested in how people respond to the external limits that may be put on their sexuality by public attitudes. There's a lot of this ooh wrinklies, ooh they can't ... by younger people, and I'm sure that must impact on older people to some extent if they're thinking of having a relationship (Older Woman, 79).

In contrast to this the researcher participants recounted from their own research practice their 'positive experiences' of researching sexuality with older people, finding the latter very willing to talk openly about sexuality. Older people did not find the topic difficult and enjoyed sharing their sexual experiences. These 'competing images' of 'negative attitudes' and 'positive experiences' could be said to be reflected in Jones' (2002) claim that there are two cultural storylines in terms of sexuality and ageing, firstly the dominant storyline of 'asexual older people' (Jones 2002:125), and secondly, the counter storyline of 'of course older people have sex too' (Jones 2002:125). The main support for the counter storyline comes from academics and practitioners (Jones 2002), which corresponds with the findings of this study. The 'competing images' however do serve to give mixed messages about whether or not researching sexuality is a relevant and important topic in which older people would consider involving themselves. It is worth noting that Gott and Hinchliff (2003:1626) found in their research focusing on the importance of sex in later life that the older participants 'welcomed the opportunity to talk about sex and discuss issues they had never talked about before.' On the one hand, views of this type from older participants involved in sexuality research could be regarded as biased, but on the other hand it could be argued that these views highlight that, for some older people, research studies may provide the only positive space to talk openly about issues of sexuality.

A number of participants made significant references to the fact that they felt that sexuality and ageing is often perceived as a sensitive topic to research, by and on behalf of, older people. The older women participants identified a range of feelings that may be experienced by other older women if they were approached to take part in such research, including feeling upset, frightened, and uncomfortable. There was a view that sexuality is a delicate topic that needed to be treated carefully and some suggestion that the word itself can create problems in terms of how older women may perceive the research.

> You've got to be careful who you send it {information about the research} to so that you don't upset people because some women over 70 would go, 'oh how dare they even suggest that I might be interested in that'. You could upset people, because 'how dare they', it's almost indecent, what you're doing (Older Woman, 75).

A difficult question to answer from the findings is whether women's perception of sexuality as a sensitive topic is solely influenced by their age. It could be suggested therefore that some older women will feel more receptive than others to involving themselves in sexuality research which may be influenced by aspects of their lives, other than their age. Therefore the more receptive older women are, the less likely they are to allow any perception of sensitivity to put them off being involved in researching sexuality. Any research which has the potential to pose a threat or incur psychological, social and financial costs to those involved can be rightly defined as sensitive research but it is important to recognize that 'it may well be that a study seen as threatening by one group will be thought innocuous by another' (Lee and Renzetti 1993:5). This variation in the perception of threat or sensitivity can also be influenced by the context within which the conversation or discussion about sexuality takes place. Although it is tempting to conclude that researchers should not assume sensitivity or difficulty at the outset of researching sexuality, Jones (2005) found that there were significant benefits to the researcher, participants and research process in framing the topic this way.

> If interviewees had not demonstrated an awareness of the sensitivity and riskiness of what they were talking about, they would have risked appearing strange, crass or rude. Similarly, if I had not displayed awareness of the sensitivity of the topic I might have appeared untrustworthy or insensitive (Jones 2005:51).

Interestingly the findings do highlight a further point involving the perception that 'other' people hold on behalf of older people, that researching sexuality and ageing is too sensitive. 'Other' people were identified as gatekeepers of health and social care services and people interested professionally in gerontology. One researcher participant highlighted a situation where the gatekeepers of a specific social networking resource were unwilling to display advertising material for recruiting research participants which used the word 'sexuality', for fear of offending the older people who used the resource. Gott (2005:63) suggests that it is important to establish 'the extent to which these concerns are the manifestations of younger people's concerns regarding talking about sex with older people', particularly if such concerns become barriers to undertaking sexuality research with older people. These feelings of sensitivity by proxy can be linked to 'negative attitudes' and in turn support the image of asexuality by silencing the voice of the older person in talking about their experiences of sexuality.

Sexuality and ageing research: What role does language play?

All the participants identified that the main issue in terms of the aspect of language within the research process centred on the concept of sexuality, its meanings and the ways it is discussed. The older women participants contributed significantly here by sharing their meanings of 'sexuality' which included sexual activity, intimacy, emotions, attractiveness, passion, identity and sexual orientation. Although the majority of the older women welcomed a definition that included more than just sexual activity, some felt it was unrealistic because of the way society's norms are imposed on the meanings of sexuality. There was a general feeling that the range of meanings sexuality held for them and other women could generate both positive and negative connotations, which in turn could influence the decision on whether to participate in research. There was recognition however that in order to undertake a broad and inclusive research study about older women's experiences of sexuality no other term was as comprehensive as sexuality.

> It means different things at different times. I mean sexuality, what other word could you put for it? I can't think of any other way you can put it (Older Woman, 75).

Sexuality is a difficult term to define, having different meanings for different individuals (Deacon et al. 1995), where the meanings are influenced by different theoretical perspectives ranging from naturalist to social constructionist (Bywater and Jones 2007). The findings therefore plausibly highlighted the task of developing a common understanding of sexuality within the research process.

Most of the participants voiced their concern about the potential for misunderstanding and miscommunication around the concept of sexuality which in turn could compromise the aims of any research study. There was an onus on the researcher to use a range of strategies that would help to develop a common understanding within the research process, such as using other terms for sexuality, reframing research questions which mirrored the terms and language being used by participants, and negotiating a shared meaning at the beginning of any researcher/

participant encounter. Heaphy et al. (1998) maintain that within their research experience negotiating on the meanings of questions between the researcher and the participant was necessary because of the complex and problematic language around sexuality and relationships. The majority of the participants favoured using 'sexuality' in a research study's advertising and information material and agreed that the use of other words to mean sexuality could lead to confusion and raise certain ethical issues. Stating the fuller definition of sexuality was also thought to be useful:

> You could put 'sexuality/sensuality' and that might make it more inclusive, but certainly emotions, feelings, relationships, identity, orientation and so on, yes I think 'sexuality' covers it. But you need to put all those words in (Older woman, 78, commenting on the possible wording of recruitment material).

Sexuality and ageing research: What are the issues in recruitment and data collection?

The findings show that some elements of the preceding macro aspects can impact negatively on the recruitment and data collection processes of research in the area of sexuality and ageing. For example, the older women participants felt that the perceived sensitivity of the research topic could lead potential participants to worry about their 'risk of exposure' if they agreed to take part in the research and that too much personal information may have to be disclosed leading to feelings of vulnerability and anxieties. Due to the possible links between 'risk of exposure' and the difficulty of recruiting participants, some of the older women participants felt that there is a crucial role for the preliminary research information to act as an important motivator for encouraging involvement in the research. Recruitment advertisements and participants' information sheets had a role in nurturing confidence and trust in the research process as well as conveying the importance and usefulness of sexuality research.

> Older women do feel that their ideas and thoughts are not being considered any more so I would think that a lot of women might jump at the idea of being able to talk about things to somebody who is going to listen to them…but they must feel that their comments and views and so forth will be taken seriously and may even somehow change things that they're unhappy about (Older Woman, 79).

Heaphy et al. (1998) identify the relevance of research to people's lives, and the wish to make an issue visible, as two of the motivators that encourage participation in research and help to build up rapport between researcher and participant. Increasing the visibility of older women's experiences of sexuality was an issue raised throughout this research and cited as the reason why many of the older women participants had volunteered. Within social work practice it is important that issues of sexuality are made more visible with a greater awareness on the part of social workers of the connection between issues of sexuality and psychosocial changes experienced by older women. Contrary to society's views it is the psychosocial changes, such as death of a partner or illness, as opposed to the biological changes, which have the biggest impact on older women's sexuality (Bywater and Jones 2007). Social workers need to be alert to these changes and open to enabling older women to raise their profile in relation to their sexuality.

The findings highlight that the important issues to consider in relation to data collection are the types of methods used and engaging older women in conversations about sexuality. Again the perceived sensitivity and personal nature of the research topic found the older women participants favouring individual as opposed to group interviews and the particular anonymity of telephone interviewing.

> Telephone interviews I think are good because you don't have a face to face and you can say things that, you know, that you can throw out.... If you're going to talk about sex or sexual activity or ... they are such deep-seated feelings about it, often feelings of inadequacy, feelings of shame, feelings of all sorts of things, and especially in our generation where sex was not something one could talk about that easily. I think that it's better to be as anonymous as possible – a voice on the phone permits you (Older Woman, 71).

Interestingly the literature supports the use of focus groups, particularly when discussing sensitive topics, because of the mutual support available from members of the group, and it is argued the group situation can provide safety to its members to discuss experiences that may not be acceptable in other situations (Frith 2000, Farquhar 1999, Kitzinger 1994). The majority of the participants recognized that many older women who would volunteer to take part in sexuality research would need some support and encouragement to be able to feel empowered to talk about their experiences of sexuality and ageing. Participants felt that there were specific ways that the research could be organized and conducted that would ensure that potential participants were adequately prepared and able to engage with the research process. Within the context of sexuality research where there are issues of sensitivity, participants' anxieties regarding personal disclosure and the complexity of sexuality, it was felt by participants that knowledge of the questions and/or areas of enquiry prior to data collection would be helpful and empowering. It is interesting to note however that a couple of older women participants felt that older women generally had the predisposition to talk freely about sexuality.

> I think a lot of women by the time they get to 70 are much more laid back, much more you know, I think we're aware of our, what shall I say, aware of our deaths and we're much more into doing things that perhaps when we were younger we would think twice about. I think we're much more daring. A lot of the women I meet are much more free I think is the word (Older Woman, 72).

Sexuality and ageing research: What is the researcher's influence?

Researchers have a pivotal role in building a professional working relationship with participants by using their skills, experience and value base to develop best practice. The older women participants felt that the researcher had a crucial role in both challenging the negative impact of the contextual issues on the research process as well as building up 'trust in the research' process starting with the recruitment strategy and following through to the task of data collection. Creating an atmosphere of trust by promising that the two ethical requirements of confidentiality and anonymity will be met is a particularly important part of sensitive research (Lee 2008) and helps to create a comfortable and enabling environment where two strangers can engage in discussions on sexuality (Frith 2000). Graham et al. (2007) in their study focusing on people's experiences of participating in research found however that ethically sound research involved more than the issues of confidentiality and anonymity. People also needed to feel valued, respected and, most importantly, feel that the researcher managed the research process in an accessible, egalitarian and competent way. An older woman participant sums up the role of the researcher by stating that

> I felt it {sexuality research} would be something I was willing to take part in as long as I thought it was done right.... I've got to feel well these people (the researchers) are doing this research, interviewing me and taking seriously what I say. I think that's important for the person that's interviewing, their attitude as well... they've got to let people see that they're very serious about their work, and that sexuality to them is a serious thing and not a sniggering thing as well, and sexuality is a big thing, it's you as a person, it's not just in the bed that's important (Older woman, 75).

Recommendations for practice

A number of recommendations can be drawn from the findings of this research study that can inform both research and social work practice in relation to older people's sexuality. Firstly, engaging with issues of sexuality and ageing needs to take place in a critical and challenging philosophical framework. For social work practice issues of sexuality need to be placed firmly within an anti-oppressive framework and social workers need to be aware of the way that ageist attitudes construct negative stereotypes of sexuality in later life. Secondly, researching sexuality and ageing needs to be undertaken within a qualitative framework so that older people are enabled to share their experiences within the context of growth, development, transformation and redefinition. Social workers are often constrained by the 'tick box' format of assessments in the questions they ask and in how it is the service user's weaknesses that need to be emphasized in order to gain resources. It is therefore important that social workers take time to encourage older people to share their experiences particularly in relation to sexuality in an enabling way. Thirdly, any discussion of sexuality with older people, be it within a research or social work context, needs to take account of society's views on sexuality and ageing. There exists a perception of sensitivity with regards to the topic in relation to research and often in relation to social work it is an issue that is easily ignored. Fourthly, the research study encouraged the use of the word 'sexuality' in a broad and inclusive sense so that all aspects of sexual expression are validated. This is particularly important when working with older people as research has found that older people are redefining what constitutes being sexual by challenging narrow definitions and embracing the diversity of sexual expression (Hinchliff and Gott 2004). Finally, the findings pointed to the fact that the researcher has a pivotal role in challenging any negative impact on the recruitment and data collection processes that may result from stereotypical views of sexuality and ageing. It is important for researchers to be aware of the contextual issues of sexuality for both the research process and the research participants. Building a professional working relationship with participants by using their skills, experience and value base to develop best practice is essential to establishing participants' trust in the research process itself and ensuring the success of any sexuality and ageing research project. It could be argued here that this highlights a parallel process for social workers when raising issues of sexuality with older people whilst undertaking assessments, and provision of care and support.

For both research and social work practice engaging with older people around issues of sexuality is necessary in order to challenge their exclusion from areas of policy, practice and research. Sexuality is central to our identity, sense of self and personhood and makes it even more urgent that the experiences and voices of older people are heard.

> I think there needs to be much more interest and attention paid to older women... we are very often invisible and inaudible so I was glad for a chance to take part in this research. Hopefully it {research} will make the general society aware ... and less hard on older women to realize that we're not just to be written off, that we're still valuable whether we have sex lives or not. We still have things to say and we still have lives to lead (Older woman, 78).

References

Biggs, S. 1997. Choosing not to be old? Masks, bodies and identity management in later life. *Ageing and Society*, 17(5), 553–570.

Braun, V. and Clarke, V. 2006. Using thematic analysis in psychology. *Qualitative Research in Psychology*, 3(2), 77–101.

Bywater J. & Jones R. 2007. *Sexuality and Social Work*. Exeter: Learning Matters.

Deacon, S., Minichiello, V., and Plummer, D. 1995. Sexuality and older people: Revisiting the assumptions. *Educational Gerontology,* 21(2), 497–513.

DeLamater, J.D. and Sill, M. 2005. Sexual desire in later life. *The Journal of Sex Research*, 42(2), 138–149.

Farquhar, C. 1999. Are focus groups suitable for sensitive topics? Edited by R. S. Barbour and J. Kitzinger, *Developing focus group research*. London: Sage, 47–63.

Fish J. 1999. Sampling lesbians: How to get 100 lesbians to complete a questionnaire. *Feminism and Psychology*. 9(2), 229–238.

Frith, H. 2000. Focusing on sex: Using focus groups in sex research. *Sexualities,* 3(3), 275–297.

Gott, M. 2001. Sexual activity and risk-taking in later life, *Health and Social Care in the Community,* 9(2), 72–78.

Gott, M. 2005. *Sexuality, Sexual Health and Ageing*. Maidenhead and New York: Open University Press/McGraw-Hill Education.

Gott, M. 2006. Sexual health and the new ageing. *Age and Ageing,* 35(2), 106–107.

Gott, M. and Hinchliff, S. 2003. How important is sex in later life? The views of older people. *Social Science & Medicine,* 56(8), 1617–1628.

Graham, J., Grewal, I. and Lewis, J. 2007 *Ethics in Social Research: The Views of Research Participants.* Government Social Research Unit: HMT Publishing Unit.

Hanley, B., Bradburn, J., Barnes, M., Evans, C., Goodare, H., Kelsom, M., Kent, A., Oliver, S., Thomas, S., and Wallcraft, J. 2004. *Involving the Public in NHS, Public Health and Social Care Research: Briefing Notes for Researchers.* 2nd edition. http:www.invo.org.uk/pdfs/Briefings%20Note%20Final.dat.pdf [accessed: 6 August 2008].

Harding' R. and Peel' E. 2007. Surveying sexualities: Internet research with non-heterosexuals. *Feminism and Psychology,* 17(2), 277–285.

Heaphy, B., Weeks, J. and Donovan, C. 1998. That's like my life: researching stories of non-heterosexual relationships. *Sexualities,* 1(4), 453–470.

Hinchliffe S. and Gott M. 2004. Intimacy, commitment, and adaptation: Sexual relationships within long-term marriages. *Journal of Social and Personal Relationships,* 21(5), 595–609.

Hinchliff, S. 2009. Ageing and sexual health in the UK: How should health psychology respond to the challenges. *Journal of Health Psychology,* 14(3), 355–360.

Hutchinson, S., Marsiglio, W. and Cohan, M. 2002. Interviewing young men about sex and procreation: Methodological issues. *Qualitative Health Research,* 12(1), 42–60.

Israel, T. 2002. Studying sexuality: Strategies for surviving stigma. *Feminism and Psychology,* 12(2), 256–260.

Jones, R.L. 2002. That's very rude, I shouldn't be telling you that: Older women talking about sex. *Narrative Inquiry,* 12(1), 121–42.

Jones, R.L. 2005. Recruiting older people to talk about sex: Some practical and theoretical reflections, in *Recruitment and Sampling: Qualitative Research with Older People,* edited by C. Holland. London: Centre for Policy on Ageing and Open University, 44–56.

Katz, S. & Marshall, B.L. 2004, Is the functional 'normal'? Aging, sexuality and the bio-marking of successful living. *History of the Human Science,* 17(1), 53–75.

Kitzinger J. 1994. The methodology of focus groups: the importance of interaction between research participants. *Sociology of Health and Illness,* 16(1), 103–21.

La Pastina, A.C. 2006. The implications of an ethnographer's sexuality. *Qualitative Inquiry,* 12(4), 724–735.

Lather, P. 1991. *Getting Smart: Feminist Research and Pedagogy Within/In the Postmodern.* London and New York: Routledge.

Lee, A. 2008. Finding the way to the end of the rainbow: A researcher's insight investigating British older gay men's lives. *Sociological Research Online,* 13(1), www.socresonline.org.uk/13/1/6.html [accessed 15 December 2008].

Lee, R.M. and Renzetti, C.M. 1993. The problems of researching sensitive topics: An overview and introduction. Edited by, R.M. Lee & C.M. Renzetti, *Researching Sensitive Topics.* Newbury Park, CA: SAGE publications.

Loe, M. 2004. *The Rise of Viagra: How the Little Blue Pill Changed Sex in America.* New York: New York University Press.

McLeod J. 2003. *Doing Counselling Research.* 2nd edition. London, Thousand Oaks, New Dehli: SAGE publications.

Minichiello, V., Plummer, D. & Loxton, D. 2004. Factors predicting sexual relationships in older people: An Australian study. *Australasian Journal on Ageing,* 23(3), 125–130.

Okami, P. 2002. Causes and consequences of a career in sex research. Edited by M.W. Wiederman, and B.E. Whitley. *Handbook of Conducting Research on Human Sexuality.* New Jersey: Lawrence Erlbaum, 505–512.

Peace, S. 2002. The role of older people in social research. Edited by A. Jamieson & C.R. Victor, *Researching Ageing and Later Life.* Buckingham, Philadelphia: Open University Press.

Perry, C., Thurston, M. & Green, K. 2004. Involvement and detachment in researching sexuality: Reflections on the process of semi-structured interviewing. *Qualitative Health Research,* 14(1), 135–148.

Pointon, S. 1997. Myths and negative attitudes about sexuality in older people. *Generations Review,* 7(4), 6–8.

Poole, H., Giles, D.C. & Moore, K. 2004. Researching sexuality and sexual issues: Implications for the researcher? *Sexual and Relationship Therapy,* 19(1): 79–86.

Pugh, S.E. & Jones, J. 2007 *Researching Sexuality and Older People.* Paper to the Social Work and Sexuality Conference, University of Salford, Manchester, 19 October.

Ringheim, K. 1995. Ethical issues in social science research with special reference to sexual behaviour research. *Social Science and Medicine*, 40(12), 1691–7.

Sanders, T. 2006. Sexing up the subject: Methodological nuances in researching the female sex industry. *Sexualities*, 9(4), 449–468.

Wahab, S. 2003. Creating knowledge collaboratively with female sex workers: Insights from a qualitative, feminist and participatory study. *Qualitative Inquiry*, 9(4), 625–642.

Chapter 4

Reflecting on Sexual Health and Young Women's Sexuality: Business or Pleasure?[1]

Michelle Brown and Priscilla Dunk-West

Introduction

The placement of pleasure within sexual health discourses is one that is problematic and often at odds with the long list of issues the sexual health worker is charged with tackling. Throughout this chapter I reflect on what gets in the way of promoting pleasure as a legitimate and sometimes political aspect to sexuality. I argue that the 'business' of sexual health is controlled by various pressures, including the need to reduce sexually transmissible infections and unplanned pregnancies. In this chapter I outline how I believe pleasure ought to fit in with the concept of sexuality as well as within educational work in sexual health. I conclude the chapter by reflecting on my professional self and how this influences the politics of my sexual health work.

The sexual health context

Sexual health is an umbrella term for organizations that provide services such as pregnancy tests, sexually transmissible infections testing, including HIV testing, as well as less 'clinical' services such as education and counselling about a range of issues related to intimacy and relationships. Although sexual health services often sit within the broad organizational context of 'health', differing professions, from medical doctors and nurses to psychologists, social workers and community workers, are employed by GUMs (genito-urinary medical clinics funded by local authorities) and non-government agencies. My experience has predominantly been working with young women both in groups as well as individually. I have, for example, provided information and support to young women accessing clinics and counselling, and through outreach settings in schools, colleges, and in the community. My roles have been varied and

---

1   An auto-ethnographic methodology (see Hayano 1979) was used to elicit material for this chapter. Though the chapter is co-written, the first person narrative was chosen to highlight that the material discussed is drawn from Michelle Brown's practice in sexual health.

have included health promotion, targeted support, education, peer education, information and advice, training and consultation.

Though my roles have been diverse, my work always involves talking to young women about their sexuality. Yet what sexuality means to individuals differs greatly. Defining sexuality in my work is not always an easy task, particularly since there are many definitions of this nebulous concept. I have used the following definition because of its acknowledgement that sexuality reaches beyond the mechanics of intimate interaction and because it helps the people I am working with better understand my work remit.

> Sexuality involves much more than just having sex. It is how we are distinguished as male and female, how we behave in response to physical sensations and how we interact in social relationships (Willynilly 2009).

The problem with the definition above, however, is that although it acknowledges that sexuality is about 'more than just having sex', it does not go far enough to identify various aspects to sexuality. Another of my preferred definitions of sexuality, which I use regularly in my sexual health work with young women, argues, that:

> Sexuality is a combination of people's sex, their sexual feelings for others, their feelings about themselves as sexual beings, their sexual orientation and their sexual behaviour (CYWHS undated).

Though they may appear too broad to concisely outline what sexuality entails, I have found that these definitions are good starting points to discussing young women's sexual health and sexuality, including whether these definitions make sense within their lives and experiences. The second definition contains a reference to 'sexual behaviour' and this is often the focus of sexual health campaigns such as those designed to reduce sexually transmissible infections such as Chlamydia or unplanned pregnancy. Yet, importantly, the definition also hints more at the affective dimension to sexual activity and I have found it a useful way to discuss pleasure and volition with young women.

Pleasure and pain

As I will explore throughout this chapter, in my sexual health work I promote discussion about sexual and relationship pleasure. For me, this means that young women not only reach satisfaction in their sexual relationships, but also are contented and choose, willingly, to be in their current relationships. I have worked with many young women who have disclosed that they have felt pressure either to be in a relationship or that they have been coerced into sexual activity. My view is that young women ought to expect to feel as equally entitled to pleasure and happiness as their partners, though this is quite a simplistic stance in many ways, it can be a useful starting point in my work.

For example, the question 'will sex hurt?' is one I have been asked by young women in various settings – in group workshops, schools, and on health promotion stalls. I have always felt it important to acknowledge that young women's feelings towards their sexual partners interact in a complex way with their own lives and, as the second definition suggests, their 'feelings about themselves as sexual beings'. Yet one answer to this question might be to talk about sexual activity in a physiological sense. This would involve reporting that, generally speaking, women take longer to become sexually aroused than men (King 1997; Weiner-Davis 2004) despite men and women having similar patterns of sexual arousal and resolution over time (see Masters and Johnson 1966). Letting young women know that it is perfectly normal to need a longer period of 'foreplay' than their male sexual partners (King 1997) – because physical arousal for a woman means a greater degree of vaginal lubrication and less likelihood of pain during intercourse – is sometimes a somewhat difficult conversation to have. Mention erections, however, and the terrain seems less risqué somehow. It is telling, for example, that very few young women talk about orgasm or masturbation for themselves, and indeed often display repulsion about that region 'down there' yet readily accept that their male partners masturbate. The term 'wanker', 'tosser' or the gesture of a male masturbating, though used in popular culture as an insult, is at least ubiquitous: there is no such reference in popular culture for masturbation in women. Given this social context, is it surprising that young women's feelings about themselves as 'sexual beings' is often peppered with the assumption that men's satisfaction is the focus of sexual interaction?

One major aspect to my work is discussing communication in relationships between young people, which often involves promoting young women's sexual agency. This can be as simple as coming from the position that sexual behaviour needs to be pleasurable for both men and women. Yet given the rise in sexually transmissible infections such as Chlamydia and high unplanned pregnancy rates, sexual health work is often overcrowded with sometimes competing agendas. Add to the mix the limited time I have with young women in some of my work settings, and the question of what specifically to focus on in the limited time I have is one I rarely feel confident I have resolved. There seems to always be more work to be undertaken. Were they not to be included in sexual health, discussions of pleasure could easily be conceptualized as barriers to the 'business' of sexual health.

To return to the question being asked by young women about whether intercourse could be painful, another perhaps more medicalized approach would be to use the opportunity to focus solely on the promotion of 'safer sex' such as condom use: this would be in line with working towards reducing sexually transmissible infections and unplanned pregnancies. Yet I would argue that there is space within sexual health work to do both. Firstly, in sexual health we can take a politically oriented approach which seeks to balance out gendered inequalities in sexual behaviour and attitudes; and secondly we can still work to reduce transmissible infections and unplanned pregnancies. This political dimension to the work both legitimizes incorporating pleasure into the core work in sexual health but also enables a critical examination of the social and individual attitudes about young women's sexuality to take place.

Offman and Matheson cite an important reason for a shift in attitudes towards women's sexual health needs. They argue that:

> Often young women's sexuality is explored not as primary, but rather as a secondary desire, that is, a response to men's sexuality (Offman and Matheson 2004:551).

Given that so much time in sexual health work is dedicated to the discussion of contraceptive choice, it is vital that considerations of 'pleasure' not only include sexual pleasure and volition but also include promoting women's agency to enjoy sexual encounters without unnecessarily being solely burdened by contraceptive responsibility. This would appear a radical undertaking since, again, the 'business' of sexual health involves educating young women about the complex and medically-oriented world of contraception.

I often wonder where is the best place to start when discussing sex and contraception with young people. Is it best to launch straight in and start off with different methods of contraception: what is available, the side effects and the associated risks of being sexually active, that is, having an unplanned pregnancy or getting a sexually transmitted infection? Although this educative approach provides young women with vital information about fertility and chemical and barrier methods to prevent pregnancy (including failure rates), is such knowledge transfer at the expense of discussions around pleasure and volition? I have found that when launching straight in with medical information I have been met with mixed reactions from young women. For example, in response to information about contraception, some tell me whether they are sexually active or not or if they are in a relationship and for how long. Tied up with such disclosures is a sense that I might be judging them; however, from my perspective it is an opportunity to model a political stance on sexual behaviour and promote pleasure-based sexual health information. Discussing relationships, for example, by separating sexual behaviour and sexual identity can help to shift dichotomous ways of thinking about same-sex attraction. Women presenting for emergency contraception, for example, are often assumed to be in heterosexual relationships when in fact they may be in same-sex relationships (Gilliam 2001). Research conducted by Eleanor Formby (2006) on lesbian and bisexual women's sexual experiences highlights the need for specific sexual health leaflets aimed at lesbian and bisexual women, or women who have sex with women, as well as relevant information about sex and relationships between women. Many women stated that they did not find it easy to find much or any relevant information about sex and relationships between women. It is important for health and educational systems to address this and to ensure that comprehensive and relevant sexual health information and education is aimed at all young women and that it does not assume heterosexuality. Not assuming identity based on behaviour can open up new levels of discussion with young women; however balancing my own agenda with the needs of young women is an ongoing task.

Research suggests that even when young people were in possession of condoms they still chose not to use them for various reasons (Holt 2002). In response to this knowledge, I, along with a colleague, developed a targeted campaign supporting young people to develop skills in negotiating condom use. During the campaign we ran focus groups with young women. A strong theme emerged that young women were not confident in initiating a conversation about using condoms if the male had not brought it up. This was usually due to how they might be perceived, for example reporting that: 'he'd think I was easy and slept around if I said I wanted to use condoms'.

A recent survey undertaken by young people in the London Borough of Sutton (Sutton Youth Parliament 2009) asked students what they wanted to learn in Sexual and Relationship Education (SRE) as well as how they preferred to acquire knowledge in these areas. The survey legitimizes the need for sexual health education, stating that 'as young people get older they will be considering using contraception and so see it as something very important to learn about' (Sutton Youth Parliament 2009: 3). The survey findings appear to reinforce the need for a broader conceptualization of sexual health than merely a focus on reproduction and medical information. Thus, the research findings support the statement that best practice sexual health and relationship education needs to highlight the importance of relationships: 78% of young people surveyed thought that relationships are an important part of SRE; however many respondents (46%) from across the school years of 7–9 (aged 11–16) said they did not think their school highlighted the importance of relationships and felt too much emphasis was placed on biological aspects (Sutton Youth Parliament 2009: 8). A further 29% said that they did not know if their schools highlighted the importance of relationships, which may suggest that the efforts by schools to explore relationships are not effective or inadequate. Such research findings not only highlight the tension I discussed earlier in this chapter between physiological or medically-based information and the political stance of the organization or individual sexual health worker, but it also raises the question as to how much agency young people have in deciding on the agenda for sexual health work. Recent Australian research with young women argues that the notion of agency is largely 'overplayed' because it fails to take into account the social factors that impinge on the choices to be made (Baker 2008, 2010). My own approach has been to take a politically active, pleasure-focused stance in the provision of sexual health services. As we shall see, sexual health is increasingly recognizing the need for emancipatory approaches to sexuality. For example, the sexual health agency in South Australia, Sexual Health Information Networking and Education (SHine SA) argues that:

Sexual health requires a positive and respectful approach to sexuality and sexual relationships, as well as the possibility of having pleasurable and safe sexual experiences, free of coercion, discrimination and violence. The sexual rights of all people must be respected, protected and fulfilled for sexual health to be attained and maintained (SHine SA 2005).

Not only is the inclusion of pleasure important to note in this statement, but placing sexual health needs within a rights-based framework allows for a more politicized approach to this area than their historically medically oriented counterparts. I will now outline what a rights-based approach to sexual health means to me and highlight key areas that I consider important areas for my own reflection.

Working with young women

I have spent a lot of time talking to young women about their rights when it comes to sex: the right to enjoy sex, to experience pleasure, to be safe and feel safe and respected by their partner, the right to say no, the right to want to have sex, and to feel free from judgement. Rights-based approaches to professions such as social work (for example, see Ife 2008) are equally at home with sexual health work with young women. This is because viewing sexual health provision through the lens of rights enables for a more politicized, active role than if I were to conceive of my work as merely responding to rising figures in sexually transmissible infections and unplanned pregnancies. Yet this politicized role is inextricably connected to my own selfhood: I am a young woman myself but I am also a feminist and committed to helping to create a society where women and men are equals.

Having a clear, feminist and political stance in sexual health does not always translate across into other roles. The following case study demonstrates how my actions and values in my sexual health work create a long-standing professional identity.

After working in the same community for a number of years and having a particular focus in one secondary school, I found myself in the school in a completely different role from my sexual health role. Susan (not her real name) was a young woman I had worked with previously in my sexual health work at the school three years ago.

I was leaving, Susan approached me. She told me that her friend needed to speak to me about something important. Since I knew Susan from my sexual health programme, I suspected it was related to my former role at this school. I agreed to speak to her friend Jane (not her real name). Jane told me she had had unprotected sex the previous night and was not sure what to do or where to go to get the emergency contraceptive pill. Although distressed, Jane was clear that she wanted to prevent pregnancy but she lacked information about how to go about doing this. After discussing the situation, I agreed to contact the nearby clinic and made an appointment for Jane to see a clinician. Still working under my work role as a 'general' worker in the school, I took Jane and Susan to the clinic where Jane would see a sexual health worker and receive the emergency contraceptive.

This example taken from my work made me question my role and my values, and helped me to realize how far my sexual health professional identity had become intertwined with me as a person. I had a dilemma: did I simply say that I was not at the school for sexual health work or did I respond to Susan and Jane in the same way I would if I were at work? From my interaction with Jane, I knew that if the young woman had to make her own way to the clinic, it would have been likely that she may not have made the appointment for various reasons. In the end, I responded as I would if I had been within my sexual health role. I provided Jane with the information she needed and I went with her to the clinic. It is this opportunistic and outreach work that tends to see immediate results in linking young people in with services and giving the relevant and appropriate information and support. The way I saw it, young women's needs do not neatly fit inside business hours. I could justify my response because I was not entering into a friendship with the two young women, even though I was out of work 'time'. The experience made me realize that I feel professionally and *personally* committed to my work far beyond what many workers would feel towards their work: I get pleasure from my profession because I do not merely see it within a business framework.

When I reflect on my identity as a community member and a worker in sexual health, I think I use my age and gender to help me in my work. Being a young woman working with young women has enabled me to reflect on my experiences and my friends' experiences, and for these to influence how I work and engage with young women. Often young women have said that they have preferred talking to someone younger than their parents, as they feel they will be listened to and not judged. As a young female professional, I have found many young women feel it is easy to talk to me and have said that they prefer talking to younger (if not younger looking) professionals including nurses and doctors. Age obviously influences the relationship a professional can forge with a young person, who may feel they are talking to a peer, and some young people may have difficulty understanding the professional boundaries with a younger professional. Yet some young people might not take me seriously, or think I am too young to be able to help them, or may get more easily embarrassed because of the lesser age difference. My response to this has been to enable young women to be supported to talk to as many professionals as possible, and to access information from many different sources.

Aside from my personal response in the case study above, the reported outcome is not always possible due to organizational constraints. Often it may seem that the 'systems' in place to deal with and support young people's sexual health and sexuality are in direct conflict with their actual needs. 'Systems' refers to the health system, the education system and to the smaller systems that exist within services and organizations. I have had experience in all of them, with a strong focus on working within the education system to educate young people about sexual health. This has seemed to be quite the contentious area, with people questioning whether the delivery of sex education is appropriate in schools, or if it should happen at home by parents and not in the schooling system. I believe that young people have the right to access information and support from wherever possible and if this can happen in the school, then it can be a positive experience. However, how sexual health education is actually delivered in schools raises many concerns and issues.

To date I have not come across a uniform and compulsory curriculum delivery of comprehensive sexual health and relationships education in schools or across countries. I believe wherever it is taught, it is important that all the facts are discussed and that young people are given enough information to make choices – information which is not value laden and judgmental. This is quite difficult to achieve, but very important. Often schools dictate what is taught to students and this is dependent on the school's attitudes, values and beliefs, along with resources available and the capacity and experience of staff to deliver the information. It seems that often education systems fail to acknowledge young people's needs and 'how best to teach' particular subjects. When young people are asked who they would like to be taught sex and relationships education by, a large percentage of students would say an expert or someone outside the school, rather than their teacher or school nurse, and this fact was also acknowledged in the survey I referred to earlier conducted in secondary schools across Sutton (Sutton Youth Parliament 2009).

As I have previously highlighted in this chapter, health systems have often focussed on statistical experience rather than educational experience. In working for a national health campaign, for example, it became evident to me that the overriding focus was on the number of people involved in the programme, rather than the education and health promotion message. This potentially had an effect on how young women responded to the programme and influenced their decisions to take part in the programme. I felt that more young women would 'eventually' participate in the programme after a strong media and education campaign that focused on health promotion and education around the need for the programme; however there were very strict targets expected, with a high number of young women expected to participate each month, which reduced the amount of education and promotion conducted and achieved. I felt that often there were young women participating in the programme without a strong knowledge of what they were doing and why. This highlights how sometimes the systems in place are limited in their impact, and how the need for outcomes can often be in conflict with the most appropriate and professional ways of practice. In this particular role I felt constrained by having to always show 'outcomes' and felt that my work was not reflective of the needs of young women. After all, isn't young women's sexuality more complex than getting involved in a national health campaign for the sake of reaching a target? This complexity, along with the pressures I mentioned earlier that a young woman faces in relation to sexual health and sexuality and the multitude of choices she must choose between, surely warrant a stronger focus than ticking a box or reaching a target.

Despite their sometimes perceived constraints and the need to reach targets, my experiences of working in and with sexual health services have generally been positive. They can provide an appropriate and professional service for young women. They are confidential, supportive, non-judgemental and flexible. Offering drop-in clinics with no need for appointments reflects their knowledge of the needs of young women, and evening and weekend clinic times additionally reflect this. I feel there is a lot of potential to improve the systems and services working with young women in relation to sexual health. Along with the challenges, however it is an ever-changing environment with new information coming to light; new contraceptive methods, new technology, and new youth cultures, all bringing with them the challenges of fitting into an organizational context in which figures legitimize service provision.

Conclusion

This reflective piece has highlighted some of the complexities inherent in my sexual health work with young women, including some of the struggles between achieving organizational targets and promoting agency in young women. I have outlined some of the barriers to the work, including social attitudes and the sometimes disjuncture between the promotion of women's pleasure and the core 'business' of sexual health. As I have argued, rights-based approaches to young women's sexualities – for example, promoting pleasure and volition – are vital values for sexual health workers to have if we are to respond to the ever shifting policies and funding of sexual health services in the coming years.

References

Baker, J. 2008. The ideology of choice. Overstating progress and hiding injustice in the lives of young women: Findings from a study in North Queensland, Australia. *Women's Studies International Forum*, 31(1), 53–64.

Baker, J. 2010. Claiming volition and evading victimhood: post-feminist obligations for young women. *Feminism & Psychology*, 20(2), 1–19.

Brauer, A. & Brauer, D.J. 2001. *ESO: How You and Your Lover Can Give Each Other Hours of Extended Sexual Orgasm*. USA: Grand Central Publishing.

Children, Youth and Women's Health Service (not dated). *Health topics http://www.cyh.com/HealthTopics/HealthTopicDetails.aspx?p=240&np=296&id=2057* [accessed: 27 February 2010]

Formby, E. 2006. *Lesbian and Bisexual Women's Sexual Health: A Review of the Literature*. Sheffield: Centre for HIV and Sexual Health.

Gilliam, J. 2001. Young Women Who Have Sex with Women: Falling through Cracks for Sexual Health Care available online at www.advocatesforyouth.org [accessed: 27 February 2010].

Hayano, D. 1979. Auto-ethnography: Paradigms, Problems and Prospects. *Human Organization*, 38(1), 99–103

Holt, J. 2002. Sex in the city: Put it on so we can get it on. Young Women's HIV Awareness Campaign. A joint project between the Women's Health Strategy Unit and the AIDS/STD Program in Darwin. *The Northern Territory Disease Control Bulletin*, 9(2), 1–2.

Huston, A.C., Wartella, E. & Donnerstein, E. 1998. *Measuring the Effects of Sexual Content in the media:A Report to the Kaiser Family Foundation*. Available at http://www.kff.org [accessed: 27 February 2010].

Ife, J. 2008. (2nd edition) *Human Rights and Social Work: Towards Rights-Based Practice*. Cambridge: Cambridge University Press.

King, R. 1997. *Good Loving Great Sex*. North Sydney: Random House.

Masters, W.H. & Johnson, V.E, 1966. *Human Sexual Response*. New York: Bantam Books.

Offman, A. & Matheson, K. 2004. The sexual self-perceptions of young women experiencing abuse in dating relationships, *Sex Roles: A Journal of Research*, 51, 9–10, 551–560.

SHine SA 2005. *SHine SA Strategic Directions 2005–2008*. South Australia: Kensington: SHine South Austratia. [online] http://www.shinesa.org.au/index. cfm?objectid=7EF44D79-E679-C8A1-8367D72F495754D6 [Accessed: 27 February 2010].

Sutton Youth Parliament 2009. Doing It in Sutton: A Report into SRE in Sutton Secondary Schools. Sutton. http://www.suttonyouth.org.

Weiner-Davis, M. 2004. *The Sex-Starved Marriage*. London: Simon & Schuster.

Willy Nilly (not dated). http://willynilly.org.uk/ [accessed: 24 February 2010].

World Health Organisation (not dated). *Gender and human rights: Sexual health* http://www.who.int/reproductivehealth/topics/gender_rights/sexual_health/ en/index.html [accessed: 24 February 2010].

Chapter 5

Growing up with a Lesbian or Gay Parent: Young People's Perspectives

Anna Fairtlough

Introduction

This chapter presents a qualitative content analysis of accounts, published in collected anthologies and magazines, by young people of having a lesbian or gay parent. It draws from life story approaches (Plummer 2001) and seeks to reflect young people's experiences from their own perspectives. It starts with the assumption that young people have rights to be heard and represented within research, policy and practice (Franklin 1995) and that they can provide unique and valuable insights about their lives (Alldred 1998, Lewis & Lindsay 2000). It then considers the insights that this analysis may offer to professionals working with these young people and their families, locating this within a discussion of UK policy and legislation.

Estimates of the number of children in the United States who have a lesbian or gay parent range from one to thirteen million (Stacey and Bilbarz 2001, Martin 1993). There are no reliable figures for the number of lesbian and gay parents in the UK. The second National Survey of Sexual Attitudes and Lifestyles in Britain in 2000 found that 2.6 % of both women and men reported having a same sex partner in the past five years, though many more reported having once had a same-sex sexual partner (National Centre for Social Research et al. 2005). Fish (2006) suggests that approximately one third of lesbians and 14 % of gay men have had children. However it is likely that many more are involved with parenting children in some capacity (Tasker 1999). The increasing visibility of such families in Western industrialized societies can be understood as part of wider social changes that show the traditional heterosexual family, headed by married parents taking specific and gendered roles, being supplemented by more 'diverse family forms with increasingly fluid and negotiated relationships' (Williams 2004:18). The gay and women's liberation movements have enabled new possibilities of 'doing family' to be envisaged and created (Weeks, Heaphy & Donovan 2001, Weston 1997). The heterogeneity, in relation to the social differences of gender, 'race' and class of lesbians and gay men has been noted (Patterson & Chan 1997, Fish 2006). Children with lesbian and gay parents also live in a diversity of family forms and situations. Some children were born to parents in a heterosexual relationship, with their lesbian and gay parent 'coming out' afterwards. Some are conceived by donor insemination and other methods of assisted reproduction. Others are adopted, fostered or raised by other relatives or friends.

Research into the experiences of children with lesbian and gay parents

When lesbian and gay parents first became visible to welfare and public agencies negative beliefs about their fitness to care for children were commonplace (Rights of Women Lesbian Custody Group 1986, Lewin 1993, Patterson 1992 & 2005). These beliefs were articulated through interlinked moral, religious, legal, and political discourses in the context of custody and contact decisions and in debates about adoption and fostering, the availability of assisted reproductive technologies and sex education. These decisions and debates were typically underpinned by assumptions about the desirability of traditional heterosexual and gendered family structures and psychological functioning. For example it was argued that children raised by lesbians and gay men would have distorted gender identities, would become lesbian and gay themselves, would be socially isolated and would suffer psychological harm. Much quantitative research in this area has tested whether these beliefs are well founded (Patterson 2005). Although this body of research has been subject to some methodological criticisms and the difficulties of researching this frequently hidden population have been acknowledged, the overall direction has been consistent: the assertion that such families are innately harmful to children has not been substantiated (Golombok 2000, Patterson 1992, 2005, Tasker 1999, Tasker and Golombok 1997).

This research has been useful in combating some of the institutional discrimination against lesbian and gay parents. The UK Secretary of State made use of it in replying to a written question about the Adoption and Children Act 2002, which for the first time permitted joint adoption by unmarried (including same sex) couples, refuting the 'possible gender confusion' of children raised by lesbian and gay parents (Smith 2002). However, as this example illustrates, some underlying assumptions have remained unchallenged. Heterosexual parenting has been taken as the norm against which other forms of parenting should be judged and measured. Deviations from 'normal' gender and sexual identities and behaviour have thus been implicitly represented as undesirable. Stacey and Biblarz (2001:176) have argued that defensiveness arising from this has obscured some real differences that have emerged in the research, and claim that children of lesbian and gay parents 'appear less traditionally gender-typed and more likely to be open to homoerotic relationships' than children with heterosexual parents. In their view these are positive characteristics. However, Hicks (2005:160) asserts that this approach is problematic too. He contends that conceptualizing gender and sexual identity as fixed entities fundamentally misunderstands the 'very complex and socially constructed sets of ideas' that he believes them to be. He calls for more qualitative, in-depth studies with lesbian and gay parents and their children in order to explore the complexity and variety of lesbian and gay life. This chapter hopes to be a contribution to the small body of such literature that is rooted in the young people's perspectives (Lewis 1980, Bozett 1987, O'Connell 1990, Tasker and Golombok 1997, Saffron 1998, Wright 1998, Paechter, 2000).

Methods

The aim of the content analysis was to explore the perceptions and meanings that the children themselves attributed to their experiences of their parents' sexuality. It draws on feminist (Roberts 1981, Stanley & Wise 1993) and other emancipatory (Robson 2002) research traditions. Central to these approaches is a rejection of the researcher as a neutral being discovering social 'facts'; rather knowledge is seen as changing, contestable and constructed in particular times and places. Such an approach requires reflexivity about personal, emotional, political, pragmatic, ontological and epistemological influences on research (Mauthner & Doucet 2003).

Responses to the stories are undoubtedly influenced in this case by the researcher's own experience of being a lesbian parent and listening to other lesbian and gay parents and their children. Years of considering these issues practically, emotionally and theoretically are a rich resource to draw on (Wright 1998). However there are some potential drawbacks of being intimately connected with the material: the researcher may be reluctant to acknowledge young people's painful experiences or negative views towards their lesbian or gay parent as this might be personally threatening or misrepresented by those who are hostile to lesbian and gay parenting. Using a research diary, reflecting with others about the interpretations and looking for negative examples, were all strategies used to enhance the value of the researcher's 'insider status' and diminish the disadvantages of this (Lasala 2000).

Life stories

A life story may be understood as an individual's account of their life that sheds light on their experiences, motivations and actions and that is set in the social world. Plummer (2001) distinguishes between the long life story, a full book length account of one person's life gathered over time, with the short life story, one usually gathered in a single interview and collected in a series. These stories are in the latter category and focus on a particular issue – children's experiences of having a lesbian or gay parent. They belong to the genre that Plummer names as the 'collective story', a genre that traces its history from slave narratives through to more recent collections of women's, lesbian and gay and other post-colonial lives. These testimonies enable people to give meaning to their lives, to affirm relationships, and to identify and counter oppression (Plummer 2001, Weeks, Heaphy and Donovan 2001). The young people make clear that telling their stories involves acts of interpreting and re-interpreting the present and the past. The published account does not represent the unchanging 'truth' but rather a particular version of events that they chose to share and construct with the person listening at that moment.

Content analysis

Content analysis describes a group of methods for systematically analysing recorded communication, including transcripts of interviews and published text (Mayring 2000). Qualitative or interpretative content analysis is used to interpret both explicit and latent meanings from texts (Reinharz 1992, Mayring 2000). Hsieh and Shannon (2005) distinguish between three types of qualitative content analysis. Two of these were used in this analysis: conventional (akin to grounded analysis), where the codes emerge from analysis of the text itself; and directed, where the codes are established beforehand through existing theory or prior research. Some initial research questions were drawn from an analysis of relevant literature, personal reflection and discussion with colleagues. A template was developed that gathered information about the source of the story, the life circumstances of the young person and particular references to positive or negative experiences of family life. This was used to generate themes in a sample of twenty stories. As these emerged, the research questions were refined and a second template to categorize the text was devised. Key categories included emotional and attitudinal responses to their parents' sexuality, their experiences of homophobia and the factors that helped them survive this, the decision about whether to be open about their family situation and the impact on the young person's identity. The data in these categories were then further analysed to identify underlying patterns. Although this proved to be a fruitful method of analysis, there was a loss in reducing these rich and often humorous, dramatic or moving accounts, so embedded in contextual meanings, to categories.

The texts analysed consist of four anthologies of stories (Rafkin 1990, Saffron 1996, Hauschild & Rosier 1999, Snow 2004) and three stories from a special edition including young people's perspectives in a magazine for lesbian and gay parents and their children (Pink Parents 2003). One anthology was specifically from children with lesbian mothers, another from children who had experienced parental divorce or separation. The accounts were published in the US, the UK and New Zealand. The texts by Rafkin, Saffron and Snow are recommended by COLAGE, a well-respected support and advocacy organization run by and for those with lesbian and gay parents, as providing valid representations of their lives.

Stories of young people aged 13 and above were used. Adolescence is understood to be a time of increasing awareness of sexuality and exposure to environments outside of parental control (Coleman & Hendry 1999). Older children and young adults would have had a breadth of experience and time to reflect on this. However this was not intended to discount what younger children had to say.

Sixty-seven accounts were analysed. Of these forty-seven were from young women, twenty from men, fifty-one had a lesbian mother, nineteen a gay father and three had both. Forty-six had experienced parental separation or divorce, thirty-one reported having a significant relationship with a parent's same-sex partner, five that they were adopted or being raised by a non-biological parent and one that he had been conceived by donor insemination.

Many of the young people did not identify themselves in terms of ethnicity and 'race'. It may be that many of these were white, adopting alongside many other white people an unquestioned assumption of the normality of being white. Four described themselves as being Black or African American and nine as having a mixed heritage, including bi-racial Black and white, Black/Greek, Hispanic/white, Chinese/white, Japanese/Irish and Maori/white. Most did not state their religious affiliation, though a significant number of the young people described themselves as Christian or as coming from a Christian background, even if they themselves were no longer practising. Two indicated they were Jewish, none that they were from another faith background.

There are strengths and limitations in using these life stories. By using accounts that had already been published the research was able to access the varied experiences of young people from a diverse range of family circumstances, backgrounds, and geographical locations. The ethical difficulties connected with interviewing children and young people were minimized as their stories were already in the public domain. These young people had already chosen to speak about their experiences. By using these sources the research was also able to draw on contacts and forms of knowledge generated by activists, practitioners and writers working with – and within – lesbian and gay communities.

However it was not always possible to ascertain from these stories how the young people were recruited, the interviews conducted and their stories written up. They may not be representative of all young people with a lesbian or gay parent. Fish (2006) examines the formidable difficulties of carrying out probability sampling with lesbian and gay populations. Little is known about the characteristics of children with lesbian and gay parents as a whole. In some crude ways this sample does reflect US findings that suggest lesbian women are twice as likely as gay men to have children and US and UK findings that between 10–14% of same sex-couples were from black or ethnic minority backgrounds (Fish 2006). These young people have elected to tell their stories and it is not known how this or other factors will have influenced what they had to say. Nonetheless, recognizing that these accounts may be partial does not invalidate them (Hicks 2005).

Findings

Young people's responses to their parents' sexuality

The stories were assigned to one of four categories: predominantly positive (thirty-one accounts), neutral (six), ambivalent (twenty-seven) and somewhat negative (three). The young people themselves distinguished their views about their parents' behaviour from their views about their parents' sexuality. For example Carla described how she had been 'hurt by my mother not because she was a lesbian, but because she loved me, and herself, so badly'. Stories were also distinguished by their length, complexity and how far the young person's responses had changed over time.

The young people in the predominately positive group reported generally positive responses to their lesbian or gay parent, to their upbringing and to their parent's sexuality. Mostly they did not express adverse reactions on learning about their parent's sexuality and, if they did, these were short lived. Although almost all of the young people identified that others' negative reactions were sometimes a problem this did not lead to major struggles or unhappiness. Fiona put it like this:

> I understood deep inside he was gay and I totally accepted it. The disadvantage
> is that others don't accept it.

Many of these young people expressed respect for their lesbian or gay parent. Lydia says about her father: 'I think that being a gay man is what made him so incredibly wonderful.' Some admired their courage in surviving anti-lesbian and gay prejudice. Randi describes how

> [...] growing up with my mother's openness about her lesbian lifestyle has
> encouraged me to become an open, honest and broad-minded person.

Others felt their parents had an enhanced ability to empathize with others, including their children. This resonates with Tasker and Golombok's (1997) findings that over one third of the young people they interviewed expressed pride in their lesbian mother. Many found their parents easy to talk to, sometimes like Rosie, comparing their families favourably to straight families that seemed 'repressed, not able to talk to each other'. Others, particularly those who had been raised always knowing about their parents' sexuality, were puzzled by other people's lack of familiarity with or antagonism to what was, for them, a normal family situation.

Some felt that their notions of family were different to children from heterosexual families and had gained extra parent(s) through their parents' lesbian and gay relationships. Like Saffron's (1998) participants, many of the young people in this group expressed positive attitudes towards what they had learnt from the lesbian and gay communities they had grown up in: they valued having an extended group of carers; found the lesbian and gay culture they had experienced to be fun; and appreciated the radical perspectives they had been exposed to, believing that this had given them a greater understanding of diversity and discrimination. What Adam valued most was 'the exposure to different types of people'.

Although some people in this group did report painful experiences within their family that arose from their parent's disclosure – for example their parents' divorce – because this had been handled well it did not leave them with lasting feelings of distress. Lydia described how she had learned from her mother that loving her (gay) father meant 'letting people be who they are, letting them go, even if that involves loss'.

The 'neutral' accounts were characterized by phrases such as 'it didn't bother me'. Their accounts were brief. They were distinguished from the first group in that they did not identify positive advantages of being raised by a lesbian or gay parent, but neither did they identify disadvantages. These young people saw their parent's sexuality as not affecting them strongly; it was their parent's business and had had little impact on their life.

The 'ambivalent' young people expressed contradictory feelings. Typically they represented their story as a journey with their reactions changing over time. Generally their accounts were longer; many gave the impression that they had struggled with some difficult issues throughout their lives. They described a range of complex family situations. Like the predominantly positive group, the ambivalent group identified many positive features of the care they received from their lesbian and gay parent; however these were combined with feelings of anger or distress that lasted some time.

Many young people described the characteristic emotional reactions to loss and change that have been identified in the literature (Marris 1991, Sugarman 1986). This was particularly true when the parent's disclosure had heralded an announcement that their parents were separating. Renee describes her reaction to her mother's disclosure like this:

> I told her it wasn't normal. I felt angry, but I was more shocked; I just had a hard time believing it. I thought that maybe it was a phase and that it would pass. Then I thought, 'now I won't be normal'.

For some the level of anti-lesbian and gay prejudice they had experienced was so devastating or extreme that despite positive feelings toward their parents, negative experiences dominated their narratives. For those who had always been raised with lesbian or gay people, the gradual realization that the rest of the world did not perceive their families in a positive way was distressing. Carey recounts how at one point in her life she began rebelling against her mother

> [...] like many teenagers do – but in another way as well. I began rejecting her identity as a lesbian – I wanted nothing to do with it.

Some identified ambivalent feelings about the lesbian or gay communities they knew. As well as the positive features identified by the first group they identified some negative ones. A few boys reported that they had heard unpleasant comments from some lesbians about their sex or felt excluded from some parts of the lesbian community. Some girls identified a contradiction in their upbringing: on the one hand they were being raised to challenge societal norms, but within the lesbian feminist community there seemed to be other norms that were also difficult to challenge. Erin felt that: 'lately he (his dad) only wants to talk about gay stuff and he's been a little self-absorbed.'

Of the three that were categorized as somewhat negative none identified positive advantages of being raised by lesbians or gay men and the young people focused on the difficulties that their parent's choices and behaviours had made for them. Two felt critical of their mother for having chosen an unstable and at times abusive partner. Another described a very neglectful mother who was unavailable to him emotionally and physically. Hence he was left vulnerable to abuse by (heterosexual) men. His was the only account (of all 67) that spoke negatively of meeting other children who had a lesbian or gay parent. However none of this group condemned their parents' sexuality per se. As Michael puts it:

> Though my mother was a lesbian, her lesbianism had nothing to do with the way she raised me. She wasn't there for me when I needed discipline or parental support … lesbianism was the excuse … but not the cause.

Experiences of prejudice and negative treatment

What came over most strongly in the young people's accounts was that they identified that the problems they experienced with having a lesbian or gay parent arose almost entirely from other people's negative views about lesbian and gay people. Fifty-nine young people gave instances in one or more of three domains: the general or institutional, the family, and peers or friends. Only four young people stated that homophobic attitudes had not been a significant problem for them. The general or institutional domain refers to the young people's experiences of living in a society where derogatory attitudes or institutional discrimination towards lesbian and gay people was routine. As Chris puts it:

> no matter how okay you are with it, there's always going to be someone who will dislike you because of it.

Wright (1998), drawing an analogy with work by McAdoo (1997) on the stress faced by black families from racism, describes this as 'extreme mundane' stress from living in a heterosexual supremacist environment. Sometimes this stress involved particular incidents: receiving threatening phone calls, being thrown out of public places, being removed against their will from their lesbian or gay parent's care, their relationship with a lesbian or gay parent being obstructed or invalidated, or their parent losing their job. Frequently it arose from the widespread use of words associated with lesbian and gay sexuality as an insult, homophobic jokes and disparaging comments about individuals and from general anti-lesbian and gay sentiments voiced in the media and in the environments they lived in. Others experienced acute anxieties for the welfare of their parents, fearing that they might be victims of violence or other forms of homophobic prejudice such as losing their job. Others felt awkward about explaining their family circumstances and feared other people's anticipated – and sometimes real – hostile, embarrassed or confused reactions.

Several young people gave instances of where judges and court welfare officers made judgments based on homophobic stereotypes. Lewin (1993) reports how lesbian mothers often used strategies of appeasement in relation to their ex-partners: for example by not applying for financial support, not challenging unacceptable behaviour or by hiding their sexuality. This was present in many of these young people's accounts. Although the young people sometimes had positive experiences of welfare professionals others had negative ones; for instance one disabled young person spoke of how his school 'helper' told him that lesbians were disgusting. Another spoke about how his social worker had presumed that his difficulties related to his lesbian parents not to the abuse he had experienced from his stepfather.

For some the hardest thing they had to contend with was their parent's own internalized homophobia. The stress of having to live with secrecy or being 'protected' from the truth was experienced as profoundly damaging. For one young man this lasted up until his father's death.

> My father, I'm 90% certain, died of an AIDs-related illness .... He couldn't even be honest about what he eventually died of.

Many young people reported homophobic behaviours from a heterosexual parent, step-parent or other member of their extended family. These included rejection, unpleasant comments, the use of religion as a weapon, and actual or threatened use of the court welfare system to limit contact or challenge custody. Frequently they occurred in the context of a custody or contact dispute. One described her father trying to snatch her and the consequent devastating effects on her own and her mother's sense of security. Michael reported that:

> My mother would say, 'of course you can love your father, even though he is a sinner and will go to hell'. As I look back I think that the message messed me up more than my dad being gay.

Many children of divorced parents have to negotiate hostility, blame and anger. However in these situations one parent appeared to abuse the power they had from being heterosexual. What the young people seemed to be saying was that the pain of living with conflict between parents and within the extended family was intensified by homophobia. The young people identified that this was damaging both to their relationship with the lesbian and gay parent and, ultimately, with their heterosexual parent.

Nearly half of the young people said that they had heard homophobic comments or experienced homophobic abuse, either verbal or physical, from other children at school or, occasionally, from other parents. Some reported being rejected by friends who had found about their family circumstances or that friends had betrayed their confidence, and this was particularly painful when it happened; however others found that friends did not reject them. In some instances the young person himself or herself was also called 'fag' or a 'lezzy' or was accused of having AIDS. Some believed that if they were seen to 'stick up' for lesbian or gay people this would arouse suspicion. This prevented alliances being made between children of lesbian and gay people and young lesbian and gay people. A few described serious physical abuse and other forms of physical harassment from peers. Like Garner (2005), these young people sometimes spoke about not telling their parents about the abuse they were experiencing. One said:

> I learnt that people could and would be cruel. I had to learn to protect my mother ...and myself from the harsh reality of the world's prejudice.

Being open

Almost all of the young people discussed the dilemmas and concerns they faced about others knowing about their parents' sexuality. As in Bozett (1987) and the Lesbian Mother's Group (1989), many, though not all, young people tried to avoid other children finding out about their parents' sexuality. Only five did not mention this at all. The young people, of course, were not able to completely control what information about their family was publicly available. In part this depended on their family structure and their parents' choices about how to represent this, and themselves, in public forums. Some parents had appeared in radio or television programmes. Public displays of affection or open acknowledgement of a same sex partner's parenting role in, for example, parent–teacher meetings meant that disclosure to others was inevitable. On occasions young people also described how their family circumstances had become the subject of gossip or rumour.

Young people made complex and nuanced decisions about what to say, when and to whom, depending on the context. Many of the situations and strategies that the young people described mirror those discussed in Goffman's (1968) classic study on the management of stigma. Sometimes these strategies changed significantly over time, with young people typically becoming more open as they moved out of middle adolescence. Decisions about what to say – in situations where they had a choice about whether or not to reveal their family circumstances – ranged on a continuum of transparency between being open in most situations to actively inventing a fictional family life. Eight of the young people gave detailed accounts of their journey from secrecy to openness. Unsurprisingly, young people's decisions about whether and what to tell were related to their responses to their parents' sexuality in general, their parents' attitudes towards being 'out' and how far they had previously experienced homophobia. Primarily, young people were concerned about what information was known about them at school and amongst peers. However some young people were also concerned, for a variety of reasons, about people in their extended family or friendship networks finding out about their parents' sexuality.

Ten of the young people were categorized as generally being open. They came over as being quite relaxed about others knowing and did not identify barriers and specific anxieties about this. Some young people experimented with telling one or two close friends. If reactions were positive then they felt empowered to tell others and to be more open. Conversely if reactions were not positive this inhibited them from telling other people.

The reasons that young people gave for feeling able to be open were both external and internal. External factors included a belief that in general people would be 'cool' about it. Particularly important was having confidence that staff at school would deal with any adverse reactions appropriately. One young person felt supported by her school's policies on equality and thought that, for example, a homophobic bully would be suspended.

Internal factors related to a positive sense of self and an understanding that adverse reactions were other people's problem, not theirs. Some young people were clear that if someone responded negatively then they would not want them as a friend. Some reported that when a relationship was important to them it was even more important for them to be honest, for example with a best friend or at the beginning of a sexual relationship. This helped them ascertain whether or not this person was somebody with whom they would want to develop a closer relationship. One young woman who was unambiguously proud of her mother as a teacher and public speaker described how she had learnt from her mother's example about the power of being open:

> 'Mother was always able to speak openly – on radio, in PTA meetings, classroom. She doesn't always get positive reactions, but she feels good about herself and what others think is irrelevant. From my mother's positive example I know that in order to be true to myself, I must be open in the world.'

A further twelve young people, though open to some, were more cautious. They reported telling a smaller number of people, usually just very close friends, and being more concerned with controlling information about their family circumstances. This was represented by the position of not 'advertising' it but not lying either. So if they were asked they would tell the truth and they would not actively try to prevent people from finding out. Though this group of young people did tell some other people about their parent's sexuality this did not mean that they always felt able to really talk about what this meant to them in a deeper way.

For those 18 young people who were categorized as being not open, stronger feelings of fear and needing to hide were expressed. These young people voiced fears that they would be rejected or persecuted if they did tell. For example one adopted girl aged 13 reported:

> I've never told anyone the real story. I don't think I will ever tell. I think if anyone found out about my mother being a lesbian, they would think us kids were strange because we have these strange mothers.

Young people used a range of strategies to manage information sharing about their family circumstances. This included: monitoring what they say so as not to inadvertently reveal their parents' sexuality, denying that their parents were gay, calling their parent's partner their best friend rather than acknowledging the reality of their relationship and inventing fictitious partners or parents for themselves. Some tried to influence their parents by asking them to remove markers such as jewellery, posters, or books that identified them as gay or lesbian, or by asking them not to show affection with a same sex partner in public. A few of the young people were angry that their parent – or more commonly – their parent's partner had refused to modify their behaviour in order to disguise their sexuality.

However, there was something of a paradox here. Where parents themselves were not open about their sexuality young people usually reported that it had not been helpful for them. It made it hard for them to find the language to talk about their family life and structure. Some parents had specifically instructed their children not to tell, either because they were concerned about their ex-spouses using it as a reason to contest custody or because they wished to protect their children from experiencing negative reactions. It is true that the young people in general wanted to have a degree of choice about how they presented themselves to the outside world. Nonetheless they reported that, while they often understood why their parent was wary of being open, this gave the message that being lesbian and gay is something that should be kept secret and therefore, implicitly, something to be ashamed of. Living with such a secret was anxiety provoking. It meant: living in fear of being 'found out'; worrying that friends would reject you if they did know or that they would be hurt that you hadn't trusted them enough to tell them; having to monitor what you said in case you let something slip and living with a sense of not being authentic or of betraying your family.

One young woman described a long journey from denial of and shame about her mother's sexuality to a position of feeling able to be open.

> Lying eroded my self esteem …. Honesty is a blessing, has helped me to reassess my values, beliefs and to value authenticity …. For the first time in my life I am experiencing connection and community around something that I had feared would always alienate me.

Summary

These findings both converge and diverge with previous research. They converge in the conclusion that children themselves do not feel they are damaged by having a lesbian or gay parent. They speak of many different experiences and different responses, both positive and negative. Fundamentally what these young people communicated was that a parent's sexuality does not determine parenting ability. Even Michael, who reported much continuing anger and distress at the enduring consequences of the poor parenting he received, did not attribute this directly to his mother's sexuality.

However this study converges from much quantitative literature in the emphasis that the young people put on the stress of living in a homophobic environment. As argued earlier, many such studies have taken the experiences of children with heterosexual parents as the norm against which children with lesbian and gay parents were compared. The starting point of this study is how children with lesbian and gay parents themselves name and understand their experiences.

Researchers have tended to conceptualize the discriminatory experiences described by these young people as 'bullying'. However there are two main difficulties with this. Firstly, the notion of bullying does not fully encompass the range of different experiences in the different domains that these young people described. Secondly, it suggests that the problem is located on an individual level, not in social, cultural and institutional attitudes and behaviours. For example, when Tasker and Golombok (1997:150) conclude that 'fear of peer group stigmatization and the experience of being bullied or teased are central elements in how children feel about growing up in lesbian mother family', they do not consider the homophobic environment that creates these fears.

Two situations made it particularly difficult for the young people to manage living in a homophobic environment. Firstly, when a heterosexual parent used homophobia to attack the lesbian or gay parent and secondly, as in Lewis (1980) and the Lesbian Mothers' Group (1989), when the young person was isolated from others in a similar situation. The study lends support to the view that children are best able to deal with homophobia or negative reactions from others when their parents are open with them about their sexuality (Lott-Whitehead & Tulley 1992, Patterson 1992). Though responses were not always negative, the young people were also clear that they wanted to decide when and how information about their family life is made public. Many reported that when support from adults was available and they knew other children in the same situation they were more able to deal with negative experiences.

Implications for practice in the UK

These children's accounts come from the US, New Zealand as well as the UK. While there are undoubtedly local and national differences between children's experiences in these different countries, some clear over-arching themes emerged in the analysis. Except for Brown's (1998) classic social work text on working with lesbians and gay men, the needs of this group of children have rarely been addressed in the British social work and social care literature. For example, a recent text (Featherstone 2004) on family support from a feminist perspective does not acknowledge their existence.

Child welfare agencies need to identify children with lesbian and gay parents who are using their services and to evaluate the appropriateness of these services. In developing non-stigmatizing services the complexities of children and young people's decision-making around being open about their family situation needs to be sensitively acknowledged. This study points to the need for practitioners to understand the varied responses that young people have to their lesbian and gay parents and the factors that interact to influence this. It is vital to appreciate the profoundly harmful effects that homophobic discrimination can have on children and young people raised in such families. It is, however, important not to assume that any difficulties that children are experiencing must be related to their parent's sexuality. Young people and their lesbian and gay parents have developed strategies and resources to support each other (Saffron 1996, Wright 1998); services can usefully learn from and build on these. Assessments and interventions need to challenge heteronormative assumptions; these children frequently describe relationships that demonstrate the transformation of intimacies (Giddens 1992) in the post-familial families (Beck-Gernsheim 1998) that scholars have discussed.

In England and Wales, as part of the changes in Children's Services brought about across the UK in the Children Act 2004, the initiative 'Every Child Matters' aims to promote an integrated response of all agencies providing services to children and their families. Two key desired outcomes of this initiative are helping children and young people to 'stay safe' and 'enjoy and achieve'. The views of children young people are intended to be central to this. This research suggests that unless homophobic practices in institutions, families and communities are combated, we are not supporting children and young people with a lesbian and gay parent to achieve these outcomes. The new Safeguarding Boards (statutory multi-disciplinary bodies charged with responsibilities for protecting children) have a real opportunity to create holistic responses to all forms of mistreatment of children based on discrimination.

Conclusion

Three landmark pieces of legislation in the UK have brought recognition to lesbian and gay people and their families: the civil partnership legislation (2005) that confers similar rights and responsibilities of marriage to lesbian and gay people, the Adoption and Children Act (2002 and 2007 in Scotland) and the Equality Act (Sexual Orientation) Regulations 2007 that outlaws sexual orientation discrimination in the provision of goods and services. Increasingly courts have been persuaded that beliefs in the unsuitability of lesbian and gay people to be parents are not borne out by the research evidence. These changes have undoubtedly made families with lesbian and gay parents more visible. It could be argued that this increasingly liberal policy framework in the UK means that we no longer need be concerned about children with lesbian and gay parents experiencing homophobic discrimination. However a number of ethnographic studies about life in UK schools (Nayak & Kehily 1997, Ali 2003, Renold 2005) paint a grim picture of routine homophobia in the children's cultures they studied. Young people themselves tell us of the importance of challenging the homophobia they experience and supporting policy changes that recognize and support their families. Only by doing so will we help remove the barriers they face to 'staying safe' and 'enjoying and achieving'.

References

Ali, S. 2003. *Mixed Race, Post-race: Gender, New Ethnicities and Cultural Practices*. Oxford: Berg.

Alldred, P. 1998. Ethnography and discourse analysis: dilemmas in representing the voices of children, in *Feminist Dilemmas in Qualitative Research: Public Knowledge and Private Lives*, edited by J. Ribbens & R. Edwards. London: Sage.

Beck-Gernsheim, E. 1998. On the way to a post-familial family: from a community of need to elective affinities. *Theory, Culture and Society*, 15(3), 53–70.

Bozett, F. 1987. *Children of Gay Fathers. Gay and Lesbian Parents*, edited by F.W. Bozett. New York: Praeger.

Brown, H.C. 1998. *Sexuality and Social Work: Working with Lesbians and Gay Men*. Basingstoke: Macmillan.

Coleman, J. & Hendry, B. 1999. *The Nature of Adolescence*. 3rd Edition. London: Routledge.

Featherstone, B. 2004. *Family Life and Family Support: A Feminist Analysis*. Basingstoke: Palgrave Macmillan.

Fish, J. 2006. *Heterosexism in Health and Social Care*. Basingstoke: Palgrave Macmillan.

Franklin, B. 1995. *The Handbook of Children's Rights: Comparative Policy and Practice*. Edited by B. Franklin. London: Routledge.

Garner, A. 2005. *Families Like Mine: Children of Gay Parents Tell It Like It Is*. New York: Harper-Collins Publishers.

Giddens, A. 1992. *The Transformation of Intimacy: Sexuality, Love and Eroticism in Modern Societies*. Cambridge: Polity Press.

Goffman, E. 1968. *Stigma: Notes on the Management of Spoiled Identity*. Harmondsworth: Penguin.

Golombok, S. 2000. *Parenting: What Really Counts?* London: Routledge.

Hauschild, M. & Rosier, P. 1999. *Get Used to it! Children of Lesbian and Gay Parents*. New Zealand: Spinifex Press in Association with Canterbury University Press.

Hicks, S. 2005. Is gay parenting bad for kids? Responding to the 'very idea of difference' in research on lesbian and gay parents. *Sexualities*, 8(2), 153–168.

Hsieh, H. F. & Shannon, S. 2005. Three approaches to qualitative Content analysis. *Qualitative Health Care Research*, 15(9), 1277–1288.

Lasala, M. 2000. When interviewing 'family' maximizing the insider advantage in the qualitative study of lesbians and gay men. *Journal of Gay and Lesbian Social Services*, 15(1), 15–29.

Lesbian Mothers' Group. 1989. A word might slip and that would be it, in *Girls and Sexuality: Teaching and Learning*, edited by L. Holly. Milton Keynes: Open University Press.

Lewin, E. 1993. *Lesbian Mothers: Accounts of Gender in American Culture*. New York: Cornell University Press.

Lewis A. & Lindsay G. 2000. (Editors) *Researching Children's Perspectives*. Buckingham: Open University Press.

Lewis, K. 1980. Children of lesbians: their point of view. *Social Work*, 25, 198–203.

Lott-Whitehead, L. & Tulley, C. 1992. The family of lesbian mothers. *Smith College Studies in Social Work*, 63, 265–238.

Marris, P. 1991. The social construction of uncertainty, in *Attachment across the Life Cycle*, edited by M. Parkes, J. Hinde-Stevenson & P. Marris. London: Routledge.

Martin, A. 1993. *The Lesbian and Gay Parenting Handbook: Creating and Raising our Families*. New York: Harper Collins.

Mauthner, N. & Doucet, A. 2003. Reflexive accounts and accounts of reflexivity in qualitative data analysis. *Sociology*, 37(3), 413–431.

Mayring, P. 2000. Qualitative Content Analysis (28 paragraphs). *Forum Qualitative Sozialforschung/ Forum: Qualitative Social Research (On-line Journal)* 1(2). http://qualitative-research.net/fqs-e/2-00inhalt-e.htm [accessed: 1 June 2006].

McAdoo, H. 1997. *Black Families*. 3rd Edition. Thousand Oaks: Sage.

National Centre for Social Research et al., *National Survey of Sexual Attitudes and Lifestyles II, 2000–2001* (computer file). Colchester, Essex: UK Data Archive (distributor), [accessed: August 2005]. SN: 5223.

Nayak, A. & Kehily, M. 1997. Masculinities and schooling: why are young men so homophobic?, in *Border Patrols: Policing the Boundaries of Heterosexuality*, edited by D. L. Steinberg, D. Epstein & R. Johnson. London: Cassel.

O'Connell, A. 1990. Voices from the heart: The developmental impact of a mother's lesbianism of her adolescent children. *Smith College Studies in Social Work*, 63(3), 281–299.

Paechter, C. 2000. Growing up with a lesbian mother: A theoretically-based analysis of personal experience. *Sexualities*, 3(4), 395–408.

Patterson, C. 1992. Children of lesbian and gay parents. *Child Development*, 63(5), 1025–42.

Patterson, C. & Chan, R. 1997. Gay fathers, in *The Role of the Father in Child Development*, edited by M. Lamb. New York: Wiley and Sons.

Patterson, C. 2005. *Lesbian and Gay Parenting*. [online]. www.apa.org/pi/lgbc [accessed: 29 January 2007].

PinkParents. 2003. *PinkParents Magazine*, 13, England: PinkParents.

Plummer, K. 2001. *Documents of Life 2: An Invitation to a Critical Humanism*. London: Sage.

Rafkin, L. 1990. *Different Mothers: Sons and Daughters of Lesbians Talk about their Lives*. Pittsburgh: Cleis Press.

Reinharz, S. 1992. *Feminist Methods in Social Research*. New York: Oxford University Press.

Renold, E. 2005. *Girls, Boys and Junior Sexualities: Exploring Children's Gender and Sexual Relations in the Primary School*. London: Routledge Falmer.

Rights of Women Lesbian Custody Group. 1986. *Lesbian Mothers' Legal Handbook*. London: The Women's Press.

Roberts, H. 1981. *Doing Feminist Research*, edited by H. Roberts. London: Routledge and Kegan Paul.

Robson, C. 2002. *Real World Research*. 2nd edition. Oxford: Blackwell Publishing.

Saffron L. 1996. *'What about the children?': Sons and Daughters of Lesbian and Gay Parents Talk About their Lives*. London: Cassell.

Saffron, L. 1998. Raising children in an age of diversity – advantages of having a lesbian mother. *Journal of Lesbian Studies*, 2(4), 35–48.

Smith J. 2002. *House of Commons Hansard Written Answers for 19 Nov 2002* (pt17). www.publications.parliament.uk/pa/cam200203/cmhamsrd/vo021119/test/21119w11.htm [Accessed 8 August 2007].

Snow, J. 2004. *How it Feels to Have a Gay or Lesbian Parent: a Book by Kids for Kids of all Ages*. New York: Harrington Park Press.

Stacey, J. & Biblarz, T. 2001. (How) does the sexual orientation of parents matter? *American Sociological Review*, 66(2), 159–83.

Stanley, L. and Wise, S. 1993. *Breaking out Again: Feminist Ontology and Epistemology*. 2nd Edition. London: Routledge and Kegan Paul.

Sugarman, L. 1986. *Life-Span Development: Concepts, Theories and Interventions*. London: Methuen and Co.

Tasker, F. 1999. Children in lesbian-led families: A review. *Clinical Child Psychology and Psychiatry*, 4(2), 153–66.

Tasker, F. & Golombok, S. 1997. *Growing up in a Lesbian Family: Effects on Child Development*. London: Guildford Press.

Weeks, J., Heaphy, B. & Donovan, C. 2001. *Same Sex Intimacies: Families of Choice and Other Life Experiences*. London: Routledge.

Weston, K. 1997. *Families We Choose*. New York: Columbia University Press.

Williams, F. 2004. *Rethinking Families*. London: Calouste Gulbenkian Foundation.

Wright J. 1998. *Lesbian Step Families: An Ethnography of Love*. New York: Hawthorn Press.

Chapter 6
Have you Heard? … Reflections on the Kerr/Haslam Inquiry

Jeanette Copperman

Introduction

There have been a number of concerns raised through inspections, public inquiries and by mental health advocacy groups about the sexual abuse of women in mental health services. In this chapter I will be reflecting on the inquiry of 2005 into the conduct of Kerr and Haslam, two consultant psychiatrists convicted for sexual abuse against vulnerable female patients which took place over a twenty-year period. Unlike other major inquiries into care failures, for example the death of children such as Victoria Climbié or Peter Connolly (Laming 2003, 2009), this inquiry received little ongoing press or professional attention.

I will start this chapter by outlining the key events within the Kerr/Haslam Inquiry and explore a number of key themes coming out of the inquiry: firstly, how professionals colluded to hide abuse and organizational silence and the implications of this for organizational culture, secondly, an examination of gender relations in the context of power inequalities, thirdly, an analysis of the professional, public and media responses to Kerr/Haslam and finally, the implications for social work practice.

Although these events took place within mental health services, they are relevant to understanding the mechanisms which contribute to organizational collusion and silence in other areas of the human services. These are relevant to ensuring that as social work moves towards full professionalization, the mechanisms which sustain abusive practices and power relations are understood and tackled. I have chosen to write about the Kerr/Haslam inquiry because it reports on an extreme example of what can go wrong. But in being extreme it tells us a great deal about everyday assumptions in organizational practices, about gender relations in organizations, violations of trust, issues in the management of the personal in the professional domain and misuses of power, which can and do take place in health and social care organizations. Further, the inquiry raises the question of how situations like these might recur and whether women would be more comfortable reporting abuse in the current climate as well as whether their concerns would be more likely to be taken seriously. In part, an answer to this relates to how the Kerr/Haslam inquiry was perceived either as a moral failing, as a feminist issue, or as a wider system failure and the role of inspection and regulation in mental health.

I have been involved with lobbying and campaigning for recognition of sexual assault within psychiatric settings and for change in the way in which this issue was acknowledged and dealt with for over ten years. I established a coalition of service users and professionals in Southwark, London and was later active in a national coalition organized by MIND that subsequently evolved to lobby and campaign on these issues. The national coalition, which engaged trade unions, professional organizations and service users, achieved many changes, not least in government policy. However there is no cause for complacency as I shall explain later on in this chapter. This chapter draws on my own experience in relation to working with these issues, including specific findings of the report and my reactions to it. The issue of 'belief' will be central to this chapter, particularly in relation to the responsibility of practitioners and professionals to report abuse. I write this chapter because I believe it raises very clear contemporary challenges for social work.

Background to the Kerr/Haslam inquiry

In the spring of 1997 a young mother went to the police in Harrogate and made a complaint of sexual assault by a former North Yorkshire psychiatrist. This was the beginning of an eight year struggle to have the truth, of what went on within the North Yorkshire Psychiatric Services during the period from 1966 to 1988 told (Haq 2006).

In 1998 after a police investigation, Kerr, one of the two psychiatrists involved was charged with four counts of rape and fifteen counts of sexual assault of women in his care. Kerr pleaded mitigating circumstance of progressive brain disease; eventually being found guilty of only one sexual assault on a 'trial of the facts'. At this point he was discharged and placed on the sex offenders register for five years. The women felt outraged by the verdict and Kathy Haq, a nurse who had been abused herself by Kerr as a young woman wrote through the police to the other women involved in the case.

> Guilt, shame and anger were words that I heard so many times as each lady contacted me …. There were also many who like myself, had thought that it had happened only to them and that no one would believe them if they spoke out. The one thing that we had in common was that these things had happened to us when we were at our most vulnerable (Haq 2006).

The women who had been abused subsequently campaigned to ensure that the truth about what had taken place was told.

The courage and persistence of the women in bringing their experience into the public domain and ensuring that effective action was, in the end, taken was recognized by the inquiry (DOH 2005) Given the range and scope of abuse which had taken place, the initial reluctance of the Department of Health to inquire into the silence that surrounded the activities of these two men for 20 years is striking. In 2004 in response these campaigns and concerns, requests for an inquiry were finally conceded, but delayed by the news that Michael Haslam, another former North Yorkshire psychiatrist had also been arrested and was now being investigated about allegations of sexual abuse by former female patients. Haslam was also convicted in 2003 on four counts of indecent assault and given a three year prison sentence. By the time the police investigations and the inquiry were complete a staggering total of sixty-seven patients had declared themselves to have been abused by William Kerr and at least ten by Michael Haslam.

The inquiry took place in 2005 incorporating cases of abuse by both psychiatrists and was one of the biggest single cases of sexual abuse by doctors in the National Health Service. Together two consultant psychiatrists had sexually assaulted at least seventy seven women in their care over a twenty year period. The Kerr/Haslam inquiry focused on three central questions:

1. How could it be that the voices of the patients and former patients of William Kerr and Michael Haslam were not heard?
2. Why were so many opportunities to respond and investigate missed?
3. How could it happen that abuse of patients, evidenced by the convictions of William Kerr and Michael Haslam, went undetected for so long?

Once the inquiry began it soon emerged that Haslam had been forced to leave Northern Ireland in 1965 following an allegation of sexual abuse by a young female. This was not dealt with at the time, resulting in his continuing to practice. More than one hundred women gave evidence to the Kerr/Haslam inquiry, either in person or in writing, exceeding those that participated in giving evidence in their court hearings. Kerr was seen as an 'outright abuser' (Kathy Haq 2009, Personal communication) and a number of the women he abused were teenagers at the time of referral to him. Women gave evidence to say that he would go as far as to suggest that they come in skirts not trousers; that he exposed himself and either raped them or forced oral sex. The extent of the psychiatrist's power emerged in the inquiry. One example was a woman, abused and made pregnant by her father, who was referred to Kerr for assistance with a termination. This request was traded by Kerr for sex. Haslam made the women believe they were having an affair with him using flattery and attention. Unscheduled domiciliary visits included unusual therapies such as full body massage with the woman naked or half naked. These practices appear not to have been questioned by colleagues as Haslam was seen as a 'guru' on sexual disorders and had published in this area (Haslam 1978). The extent of his arrogance was noted during the inquiry. Whilst in prison for sexual assault he threatened women who gave evidence against him with libel suits. The Inquiry sought that the government indemnify the women before many would give evidence (Pleming 2009, Personal communication). Kathy Haq also noted that the women's medical records had notes made to discredit them should they should try to raise the alarm (Haq 2009, Personal communication). Both men would make appointments at the end of each working day with women, in remote parts of the hospital. One nurse related to the inquiry her loss of career as a result of raising her concerns with the matron at the time, who responded by calling her a 'dirty young woman' and blaming her for the abuse. (Haq 2009, Personal communication)

Through its power to summon witnesses, the Kerr/Haslam Inquiry gathered evidence from doctors, nurses, social workers and former hospital managers who had remained silent:

> We sat and listened as (they) gave their evidence and in many cases excuses as to why, even though they admitted they were aware of a 'problem', they did nothing. The words 'I cannot recall' or 'have no recollection' must have been the most widely repeated of all throughout the inquiry hearings .... (Haq 2006)

As the inquiry painstakingly traced the complaints the women had made back to those they had complained to, they discovered that some General Practitioner surgeries had heard frequent complaints from different women over a period of time but failed to take action, citing the individual women's reluctance to take the case further as justification.

That this abuse and betrayal of trust often had long lasting consequences for the women who had experienced them is well established. (CHRE 2009, Richardson et al. 2008) Acts of suicide following abuse were reported amongst the women abused by these two men (Haq 2009, Personal communication) chiming with my own knowledge and anecdotal evidence when campaigning on this issue in the 1980s and 1990s.

Recommendations of the inquiry

The Inquiry Report contains seventy four recommendations to prevent future sexual abuse and guidelines for dealing with abusing health care professionals more swiftly. It highlighted existing flaws in complaints procedures within the National Health Services as well as raising organizational and cultural issues and the importance of support for patients making complaints. A national prevalence survey was recommended to:

> show the prevalence of sexual assaults, sexual contact, or other sexualized behaviour, between doctors and existing and/or former patients – particularly in the field of mental health.'(DOH 2005: chapter 30)

Despite a response from the government and relevant professions, many of the recommendations have yet to be fully implemented. To date no national prevalence survey has been conducted. Recommendations that doctors and nurses be given better training on handling complaints and the provision of independent advocacy to all patients, particularly female psychiatric patients in reporting abuse, is still not consistently being carried out.

In her response to the report, Kathy Haq stated:

We know how difficult it is to speak out when you have been sexually abused and certainly we agree with the need to have someone independent to support a complainant, someone who is trained in that field. This, for us I believe, is the most important of the recommendations made .... If they (the women) had been supported by someone who would have 'stood up for them' then they would have followed it through (Haq 2006).

Themes from the Kerr/Haslam inquiry

Professional collusion with abuse

It is challenging to put ourselves into the shoes of practitioners and managers confronting the power of these two psychiatrists, Kerr and Haslam. A counsellor, a social worker and a psychologist were amongst those who received complaints and failed to take effective action. Issues within the practice culture of the North Yorkshire National Health Service at the time were noted to include poor record-keeping; lack of accountability of professionals; management failures; disbelief of the women; lack of support for expressions of concern and complaints; and disproportionate power wielded by the consultants in a hierarchical environment.

The inquiry noted a tolerance that appeared to have developed amongst some of the General Practitioners to psychiatrists having sexual relationships with patients in their care. This was common knowledge amongst health professionals but subsequently disparaged and trivialized. This attitude is evidenced by the way in which Haslam, who had been forced to retire (with thanks) from his post in the National Health Service, was allowed to work out his notice with no restrictions on his activities. He was also given a reference which enabled him to continue to work in the private sector for a further three years. The reluctance to act on the part of higher management when abuse was brought to their attention, whilst known about at an informal level, meant that 'turning a blind eye' created a culture of impunity for predators. The combination of these barriers to complaining and reporting abuse included staff being unclear whom to report abuse to or how to take this further; a trivialization of sexual harassment and abuse and in some cases active discouragement by one or two General Practitioners from seeking redress. The profound emotional impact of being abused by someone with a duty of care whilst vulnerable was completely underestimated. Such lack of understanding of the seriousness of these invasions all combined to make reporting difficult.

There were also failures to connect together different instances and reporting of abuse and exchange information. Many of these themes figure in other instances of institutional abuse and the misuse of power such as those in the Jersey Children's Home and the North Wales Children's Homes (DOH 2005, Stanley et al. 1999).

Particular barriers noted by the inquiry included lack of belief by professionals about the assaults, based on women's psychiatric histories, even though these did not indicate any history of fabricating accusations. Many women were referred originally for anxiety and depression with no connection to delusional thought. Therefore many women lacked the confidence that they would be believed and the support to take it further.

The role of gossip and rumour

Much of what was known at the informal level in the organization was not acted upon at the formal level. For example many of the General Practitioners decided at an informal level not to continue referring female vulnerable patients to Kerr and Haslam yet took no formal action to stop their activities. The literature on organizational silence might give some clues as to why information well known at the informal level is not acted upon within the formal level and the factors which contribute to this (Henriksen and Dayton 2006).

Whistleblowing

Lin Bigwood, a nurse did speak out and raised repeated concerns over a five-year period following a report from a patient about her sexual relationship with Kerr during clinical history-taking. Her career suffered as a result of such whistleblowing. The Public Disclosure at Work Act (1998) and subsequent case law has strengthened support and protection for whistleblowers. However as Pleming reflects from his experience of conducting the Kerr/Haslam inquiry 'It is difficult to be a whistleblower at every level, you have to encourage the isolated whistleblower to be part of the culture of the place (to raise malpractice), otherwise they in turn can become a victim, that is why culture change is so important'. (Pleming 2009, Personal communication) A common feature of inquiries into abuse such as the inquiry 'Lost in Care' into abuse within North Wales children's homes (Waterhouse 2000) and the 'Bristol Babies' inquiry (Kennedy 2001) is that there is often an individual who has tried to raise the alarm several times and their career suffers as a result and they become marginalized with their organization.

Achieving culture change

Sexual misconduct or boundary violations are complex. Pleming (2009) suggests that these range from romance to rape and challenge the professions to debate what and what is not acceptable; to clarify training required and to address culture change. He warns about 'grooming processes' with vulnerable women (Pleming 2009, Personal communication).

Determining policy and ethical principles in this area needs to start with a careful definition of what should be the proper boundaries between professional and patient. In doing so, a difficult balance needs to be struck – allowing professionals to show patients empathy, respect, support and reassurance, but ensuring that this remains within the proper boundaries of the relation between professional and patient and does not risk an inappropriate and possibly damaging emotional attachment on either side (DOH 2005:28).

Responses to the Kerr/Haslam inquiry

The government response to this and two other inquiries, that of Harold Shipman (Smith 2005), who was responsible for murdering his patients, and Ayling, another doctor who abused women in his care (Pauffley 2004) resulted in the White Paper 'Trust Assurance and Safety – the regulation of health care professions'(DOH 2007). The healthcare regulatory authority was set up, drawing up detailed guidance for the health professions and information for patients about their rights, although this has not been widely publicized (CHRE 2009). Codes of professional practice have been issued to clarify what might have been previously regarded as an unclear situation to take action on abuse (CHRE 2009). Legislation on sexual misconduct has also been strengthened via the Sexual Offences Act (2003) and the Mental Capacity Act (2005), which makes it a criminal offence to have sexual relations with a vulnerable patient.

In relation to policy, 'Mainstreaming Gender: A Women's Mental Health Policy' (DOH 2002) and the Implementation Guidance that goes with it (DOH 2003) have introduced, amongst other things, a duty to appoint a person responsible for gender equality in each health care trust. Trusts also have a duty to implement policies on privacy and dignity and choice, including the provision of women only facilities; provision of training for staff on understanding and talking about violence and the other power dynamics which inform women's lives (DOH 2003) The Clear Boundaries Project was established to clarify norms and procedures for relevant professions. It certainly would not be possible for General Practitioners to act in the way that they did in Harrogate. Routine clinical governance has also been strengthened. Previously there has been no single guidance within the National Health Service on sexual misconduct. The 'No Secrets' guidance directed to the multi-agency protection of vulnerable adults (DOH 2000) now clarifies professional responsibilities where there is suspected abuse of vulnerable adults and can be used in relation to suspected abuse.

Legislation and policy to support whistle blowers has been strengthened in the Public Interest Disclosure Act (1998) and subsequent case law. Despite these developments there is no cause for complacency. Every survey of mental health settings before and since Kerr/Haslam continues to reveal sexual assault and abuse and ongoing barriers to effective action.

For example, the Health Observatory found in a snapshot survey in 2005, the same year as the published Kerr/Haslam inquiry, that there were 122 reported sexual assaults and 19 reported rapes in mental health settings between 2003 and 2005 – 11 were alleged to have been from staff. There were three unwanted pregnancies reported, 19 cases of exposure, 18 of sexual advances and 26 of touching (NPSA 2006). The Department of Health initially tried to hold back the publication of the information. Louise Appleby subsequently issued a statement casting doubt on whether 13 of the 19 rapes were genuinely rapes (Appleby 2006). It is unclear on what basis the DOH reached this conclusion, presumably partly on whether the Crown Prosecution Service would be likely to take the cases forward – however the Kerr/Haslam report warns precisely against using such criteria when determining whether a serious event has taken place, given the culture of disbelief of female psychiatric patients. In conclusion, it remains difficult for individual isolated women to take a complaint forward. In response to the Kerr/Haslam's recommendation for advocacy, organizations such as Public Concern at Work, and Witness, an organization working specifically around abuse by health and social care professionals by providing training, advocacy and support to victims, were established, However the latter organization no longer receives core funding for its work.

Gender relations and Kerr/Haslam

One way to understand the Kerr/Haslam events being not widely discussed is within the context of gender relations and mental health. The last thirty years have seen a considerable amount of lobbying, campaigning and research on these issues (Barnes et al. 2002, Perkins et al. 1996). The gendered dimension of the abuse – male doctor on female patients in Kerr/Haslam – was articulated in the inquiry report; however professional responses to the inquiry have not highlighted gender. The response of the Royal College of Psychiatrists, for example, makes little mention of the gender dimension of the abuse that took place issues (RCP 2007), although surveys of psychiatrists show a clear gender dimension in those likely to abuse (Fahy 1992). It is difficult to see how culture change can take place if gender is ignored as a key factor in understanding sexual assault/abuse. The ability of mental health services to work with gender perspectives and to listen to the views of women generally has long been a concern (Williams 2005). Mainstream mental health services have been and remain dominated by individualized and medicalized approaches to mental distress within which social perspectives remain marginalized (Barnes et al 2002, Williams et al. 2001). The battle to gain even the most basic physical security for women in psychiatric inpatient wards over the last twenty years testifies to the difficulty that feminists, users and voluntary organizations, researchers, committed practitioners and managers, have had in changing mainstream mental health practice (Goodman 2005, MIND 1994, Perkins et al. 1996, Resisters 2002).

Relational safety

Many studies identify having someone to talk to and who is available to listen as vitally important. Women service users involved in a study by Cutting and Henderson (2002), for example, reported that staff were inaccessible, a frustration when they wanted someone to talk to. Trusting supportive relationships are key to creating safer environments. Research evidence also suggests that rape, sexual harassment and threats have been for some time and remain significant concerns for women inpatients (Copperman and Mc Namara 1999, Williams et al. 2001) and have a significant impact on women and their recovery. Concerns emerge repeatedly when general surveys of inpatient settings are carried out. For example, a UK survey in 2001 found a significant level of concern about safety in services – 29 respondents (30.21%) were concerned about the lack of safety in current service provision. (Williams et al. 2001). Reports and studies from the US and the UK show that harassment and assaults are perpetrated by staff as well as other patients and in a variety of settings (Bouhoustos et al. 1983, DOH 1992). One hospital study in the US found that 71% of patients had been threatened with physical violence, 38% had been sexually assaulted and 27% had been sexually assaulted by staff (Nilbert et al. 1989). In 2004 as part of their 'Ward Watch' campaign, MIND surveyed current and past inpatients about their experiences of staying on a psychiatric ward. Their findings show that whilst improvements have been made, there are worrying trends which need to be addressed. Of the 338 responses, 23 % said they had been admitted to mixed sex accommodation. The survey found that a third of respondents did not have access to single sex bathroom facilities and two-thirds did not have access to single sex daytime facilities. Just under a third reported feeling unsafe in hospital and 51% percent of respondents had experienced being verbally or physically threatened during their stay. Sexual harassment was experienced by 18% percent of respondents and 5% percent reported sexual assault. Racial harassment as well as harassment on the basis of an individual's sexuality was also reported (MIND 2004).

Women's sexuality in mental health settings has also been viewed as problematic. For example one study found that 'sexual acting out' was mainly applied to women in mental health settings although there is ample evidence of inappropriate sexual behaviour from men (Copperman 1989). Broverman et al. in their study of mental health professionals' attitudes also found that it was impossible to be a mentally healthy woman and a mentally healthy adult (Broverman et al. 1970). I would argue that culture change needs to encompass a view of the gendered power relations found in organizations in order to tackle the spectrum of sexual harassment and assault.

Public and professional knowledge about Kerr/Haslam

Pleming noted that it was 'stressful' to conduct the inquiry (Pleming 2009, Personal communication). Certainly the reports of abuse by the women, and their accounts of repeated attempts to get heard, make difficult reading. The recommendations of the report are directed to government, to the professions, to regulators, to educators, to managers and to practitioners; yet many of these groups remain largely unaware of it. This raises issues about how difficult knowledge is kept in the public sphere when it is challenging to the mainstream and awkward to face. This has been an ongoing concern for feminists working in the sphere of violence. It is tempting to think that perhaps this silence exists because it was a one-off, an aberration that took place in an isolated part of North Yorkshire from the 1960s to the 1980s, and that such events could not be repeated. We have moved a long way since the 1980s in terms of policy and legislation. But the lack of public outcry and silence which surrounded the inquiry and the continuing lack of open discussion of sexual harassment and abuse in mental health settings is a cause for concern. It raises questions about public and professional understanding of these issues.

Given that the inquiry's brief was to examine the silence and inaction around the activities of these two psychiatrists, it is surprising that this lack of knowledge includes mental health managers, policy makers and experienced mental health practitioners. It is also striking how little interest it has evoked in public discourse with a few honourable exceptions. This contrasts with the high profile of other inquiries referred to earlier (Laming 2003, 2009, Waterhouse 2000, Kennedy 2001), given the complete lack of media coverage and public response.

Dilemmas from the perspective of a manager

Sue Waterhouse, National Equalities Advisor, has contributed her reflections on some of the dilemmas she has encountered in this area following on from her experiences as a mental health manager. She gives insights into why at the time some practices seem to go unchallenged. One issue she identifies is the role of intuition and how to ensure suspicions come to light without unfairly accusing a colleague:

> Over my years of working in mental health services the lack of awareness of the potential for staff to abuse service users has been evident. Where there has been concern, staff have found it difficult to raise it. Staff, particularly in the more disturbed environments, have historically be taught and encouraged to trust and rely on their colleagues. After all this is what good team working is all about. To then suspect a colleague of abuse goes against the grain. Abuse is often concealed, if a team member suspects a colleague of abuse there is often not a lot of information to go on. It would be usual if you have suspicions to discuss them with others, but in the case of a colleague it is difficult for an individual to risk voicing these concerns in case they are wrong.

She reflects on an instance when she had concerns about a colleague but it was only when she and a number of female colleagues got together that they were able to trust their intuition:

> On reflection my suspicions were raised by his general demeanour with female service users. He generally was too ingratiating with young women who largely had a history of sexual abuse in childhood. He regularly tried to win their favour by overstepping boundaries and giving them special treatment. Whilst I was suspicious, there was nothing concrete to act on… I thought I was the only person who had these thoughts, as he seemed to get on well with the rest of the team.

> After a few months, in a social situation with several other female colleagues one of my colleagues mentioned that she was convinced that he would at some point rape a female patient. This seemed to be an extreme view but mirrored my fears exactly. Once this had been spoken several of the other colleagues stated that they had similar thoughts. Nobody could pinpoint what exactly it was about this person that caused such an extreme reaction in all of us.

Although he left at the time he was rehired later on, warnings were ignored and the staff member went on to be convicted of a sexual assault on a female patient.

As a manager Waterhouse had had to challenge staff when they dismissed a reported sexual assault without investigation and as a manager she had also faced grey areas such as dealing with sexual relationships between colleagues in unequal power positions (Sue Waterhouse 2009, Personal communication).

Why discuss Kerr/Haslam in the context of social work?

Sexual misconduct is an ongoing issue in professional practice for both the social work and health professions. The GSCC conduct committee has dealt with 24 cases where social workers were alleged to have been involved in sexual relationships with service users; this has represented approximately 40% of their case load (Carson 2009). Following these investigations, 15 social workers were removed from the register, five were admonished and four were suspended. The Council for Health Care Regulatory Excellence (CHRE) from January 2005 heard 274 cases of sexual misconduct. Of these, 156 practitioners were removed from the register of health professionals, 26 were suspended and 25 were maintained but with conditions attached (Carson 2009).

The Inquiry noted that the work of organizations such as Witness showed that sexual or other abuse of patients by health professionals is more frequent than previously supposed, and that broad estimates in other countries suggest that the prevalence could be as high as 6–7% of health professionals (DOH 2005). In some cases, abuse can initially manifest or be disguised as a minor infringement of the proper 'boundaries' of trust which should exist between professional and patient, and then progress imperceptibly to more serious abuse. For this reason, it is now common to treat abuse as an extreme form of 'boundary transgression' (DOH 2007:54–61).

Many cases in both the GSCC and the CHRE's caseloads have related to male practitioners and vulnerable female service users, including mental health clients. There is robust evidence of consistent underreporting of abuse amongst this group and we can assume that the actual cases which take place are more numerous. Professional attitude surveys reveal confusion over what constitutes safe ethical practice. When Community Care surveyed social workers in 2008, they found that whilst 70% of social workers felt that sexual relationships with service users were never acceptable, 14% said they were acceptable, at least sometimes, and a further 16% said they were unsure (Carson 2009). This confusion and the current lack of clear guidance to accompany the social work code of practice is worrying given the amount of power that social workers have over vulnerable service users. Social work itself now has a regulatory body; the General Social Care Council. The profession has codes of guidance (GSCC 2002) and the means of disciplining and striking off erring professionals; none of this was available in the 1980s. However it has yet to develop clear detailed guidance on the issue of sexual boundaries and misconduct as the health professions have. In addition Public Concern at Work expressed concern that the social care sector is a 'long way behind even the health service' when it comes to supporting whistleblowers (Community Care 2005).

Conclusion

There can be an assumption that because we are working in the public sector, sufficient checks and balances are already in place, and it is largely in the private sector that people are vulnerable. However experience shows that this is not the case, that organizational cultures which are not open to scrutiny, which ignore gender and power relations and are not able to talk about sexuality can make the reporting and investigating of abuse hard to take up. This challenges us to think about how we formulate effective interventions to oppressive organizational practices and how we as individuals make choices not to remain silent bystanders to abusive practices even when there are personal costs. It raises questions about how we find the confidence as professionals, activists and users to speak out about abuse and how we work together to make sure that our concerns are taken seriously.

Both my own experience and the inquiry report emphasize that culture change to accompany policy and guidance is also crucial. From my point of view there is still a good deal to do on that, both in practice and in training. The remedies are not only technical and professional and to do with the criminal justice system, although they are that too, but also to do with women taking power and speaking to each other about these issues. In Sue Waterhouse's example, it was at an informal level that women were able to exchange information initially about a dangerous practitioner and trust their intuition. Discussion, organizing and advocacy are key to successful prevention. As an isolated individual it can be difficult to trust your intuition and take action, and the costs can be great to the individual. The creation of supportive networks of professionals, users and activists to help identify and stop the trivializing of abuse is crucial.

Standard setting, regulation and managerial responses also need to be situated within a context of violence against women. It means staying with knowledge that is uncomfortable knowledge within organizations, and this will carry risks. This knowledge will be resisted, violence and abuse are hard to look at and one organizational response is to codify and then put the knowledge aside. As Menzies-Lyth (1959) points out in her work on organizational defences against anxiety, a focus on tasks and procedures can be a defence against anxiety. In this context procedures need to be backed up with real power, understanding and action.

Never Again?

Nigel Pleming QC, who conducted the Kerr/Haslam inquiry suggests three starting points in relation to prevention in the future:

1. Acknowledge that sexual contact happens – it happens to approximately 7% of patients and it is important to start from that assumption. There needs to be serious discussion in the professions about where the boundaries are.
2. Acknowledge that if you are not doing it yourself it is likely that one or two colleagues are, so you have to be alert to the signs/things that you hear from patients. You have to be clear that when you do have information you have to pass it on and what the channels are.
3. Build such issues into professional training. Ensure every library has a copy of the Kerr/Haslam report, ensure all health and social care students receive one session on every health and social care training about establishing clear boundaries and also on the duties to report suspected abuse.

(Pleming 2009, Personal communication)

Some final words for social workers

As well as the recommendations that Pleming makes for training, awareness and action, I would argue that to bring about culture change we also need sustained effort to create environments where women discuss these experiences and challenge abusive practices. Our ideas about sexuality, what is and is not acceptable are arrived at through discussion and debate and it is crucial that the feminist voices of professionals, users and activists are present in these discussions within the social work arena. I believe that there are aspects of social work knowledge and practice which are important to supporting ongoing culture change. I would argue these are important to future prevention. In my view these are:

- A critical engagement with social policy and in the policy making arena within social work and outside of it from a position of foregrounding gender relations and power inequalities.
- A focus on social perspectives in mental health. This encourages us to situate women's mental health within the context of their lives and in turn helps us to be sensitive to backgrounds of trauma and abuse and the implications of that for future vulnerability.
- Highlighting our radical tradition of community action, which emphasizes independence in organizations and cultures of resistance and challenge to mainstream ideas and practices. I would like to see us foreground the social work/community work traditions of network building, social inclusion and social action. These strands of social work are not just as part of our history

but as part of our present can help support culture change.
- Supporting and understanding the value of independent advocacy. Independent organizations like Witness and rape crisis centres need ongoing support. Women prefer independent organizations to discuss experiences of sexual assault where they are not pathologized.
- Finally valuing our experience and training on listening to difficult experiences and reflecting on our own reactions.

I now work within an interprofessional context. The particular contribution that social work can make in an interprofessional environment to understanding and working with the voluntary sector is noticeable. Perhaps because we have arrived at professionalization later than other professions we have more experience of coalition building with grass roots organizations and the voluntary sector. Activists, service users, concerned managers and professionals helped by sympathetic politicians and journalists achieved a change in government policy. We can aspire now to create environments where when women speak out they are never again dismissed. We owe this much at least!

I wish to acknowledge the personal discussions I had with Kathy Haq, Nigel Plemming Q.C. and Sue Waterhouse from the National Mental Health Development Unit which I found valuable when writing this chapter and thank them for the time they gave me. The views in this chapter are expressly my own and should not be attributed to others.

References

Appleby, L. Quoted in Hussain, A. 2006. Most alleged rapes of psychiatric patients almost certainly never happened http://www.Pschychminded.co.uk [Accessed on October 16th 2009].

Barnes, M., Davis, A., Guru, S., Lewis, L. & Rogers, H. 2002. *Women – Only and Women – Sensitive Mental Health Services: An Expert Paper:* Final Report to the Department of Health: Unpublished.

Bouhoustos, J., Holroyd, J., Lerman, H., Forer, B. & Greenberg, M. 1983. Sexual intimacies between psychotherapists and patients. *Professional Psychology: Research and Practice*, 11(3/4), 425–464.

Broverman, I.K., Broverman, D.M., Clarkson, F.E., Rosenkrantz, P.S. and Vogel, S.R. 1970. Sex role stereotypes and clinical judgement in mental health, *Journal of Consulting and Clinical Psychology*, 34(5),1–7.

Carson, G. 2009. GSCC may issue guidance on sexual boundaries with users, *Community Care Magazine* 1st June. www.communitycare.co.uk [accessed 1 March 2010].

Community Care, 2005. Are social workers protected when they blow the whistle? *Community Care*, 3rd February 2005. www.communitycare.co.uk [accessed 1 March 2010].

Copperman, J. 1989. *Sexual Abuse of Women in Psychiatric Hospital*, MSc Thesis Unpublished.

Copperman, J. & McNamara, J. 1999. Institutional abuse in mental health settings: survivor perspectives, in *Institutional Abuse: Perspectives Across the Life Course*, edited by N. Stanley, J. Manthorpe & B. Penhale. London: Routledge.

Council for Healthcare Regulatory Excellence. 2009. *Clear Sexual Boundaries between Healthcare Professions and Patients: Information for Patients and Carers*. London : CHRE.

Cutting, P. & Henderson, C. 2002. Women's experiences of hospital admission *Journal of Psychiatric and Mental Health Nursing*, 9(6), 705–712.

Department of Health. 1992. *Report of the Committee of Inquiry into Complaints about Ashworth Hospital*, Volume 1. London: HMSO.

Department of Health. 2002. *Women's Mental Health: Into the Mainstream*. London: Department of Health.

Department of Health. 2003. *Mainstreaming Gender and Women's Mental Health: Implementation Guidance*. London: Department of Health.

Department of Health. 2005. *Kerr/ Haslam Inquiry: Full Report*. London: The Stationery Office.

Department of Health. 2007. *Safeguarding Patients: The Government's Response to the Recommendations of the Shipman Inquiry's Fifth Report and to the Recommendations of the Ayling, Neale and Kerr/Haslam Inquiries*. London: The Stationery Office.

Department of Health and Home Office. 2000. *No Secrets: Guidance on Developing and Implementing Multi-agency Policies and Procedures to Protect Vulnerable Adults from Abuse*. London: The Stationery Office.

Fahy, T. 1992. Sexual Contact between Doctors and Patients, *British Medical Journal*, 304, 1519–1520.

General Social Care Council. 2002. *Codes of Practice for Social Care Workers and Employers of Social Care Workers*. London: GSCC.

Goodman, J. 2005. *A User's Perspective – Working for Change and Improvement in Services for Women in Southwark*, http.//www. scie.org.uk. [Accessed 29 February 2010].

Haq, K. 2006. *The Kerr/Haslam Inquiry: The Women's Story*. London: Witness Against Abuse.

Haq, K. 2009. Discussion on Kerr/Haslam Inquiry (Telephone Communication, 28th September 2009).

Haslam, M.T. 1978. *Sexual Disorders: A Practical Guide to Diagnosis and Treatment for the Non-Specialist*. Tunbridge Wells : Pitman Medical.

Henriksen, K. & Dayton, E. 2006. Organizational silence and hidden threats to patient safety. *Health Services Research*, 41(4), 1539–1554.

Kennedy, P. 2001. *Bristol Royal Infirmary Inquiry*. London: The Stationery Office.

Laming, H. 2003. *Report of the Victoria Climbié Inquiry.* London: The Stationery Office.

Laming, H. 2009. *The Protection of Children in England: A Progress Report.* London: The Stationery Office.

Menzies-Lyth, I. 1959. The functions of social systems as a defence against anxiety: A report on a study of the nursing service of a general hospital', *Human Relations,* 13, 95–121; reprinted in *Containing Anxiety in Institutions: Selected Essays, vol. 1.* Free Association Books, 1988, 43–88.

MIND. 1994. *Stress on Women: Policy Paper on Women and Mental Health.* London: MIND.

MIND. 2004. *Wardwatch: Mind's Report on Hospital Conditions for Mental Health Patients.* London: MIND.

National Patient Safety Agency. 2006. *With Safety in Mind: Mental Health Services and Patient Safety (Patient Safety Observatory Report 2).* London: National Patient Safety Agency.

Nilbert, D., Cooper, S. and Crossmaker. 1989. Assaults against residents of a psychiatric institution: residents' history of abuse. *Journal of Interpersonal Violence,* 4(3), 342–349.

Pauffley, A. 2004. *The Ayling Report.* London: The Stationery Office.

Perkins, R., Nadirshaw, Z., Copperman, J. & Andrews, C. 1996. *Women in Context: Good Practice in Mental Health Services for Women.* London: Good Practices in Mental Health.

Pleming, N. 2009. *Leading the Kerr/Haslam Inquiry* (Telephone Communication, 16th October 2009).

Resisters. 2002. *Women Speak Out: Women's Experiences of Using Mental Health Services and Proposals for Change.* Leeds: Resisters.

Richardson, S. Cunningham, M. et al. 2008. *Broken Boundaries: Stories of Betrayal in Relationships of Care.* London: Witness Against Abuse.

Royal College of Psychiatrists. 2007. *Sexual Boundary Issues in Psychiatric Settings.* London RCP. www.rpscyh.ac.uk [accessed:15th September 2009].

Smith, J. 2005. *The Shipman Inquiry.* London: The Stationery Office.

Stanley, N., Manthorpe, S. & Penhale, B. (editors) 1999. *Institutional Abuse: Perspectives Across the Life Course.* London: Routledge.

Waterhouse, R. 2000. *Lost in Care: Report of the Tribunal of Inquiry into the Abuse of Children in Care in the Former County Council Areas of Gwynedd and Clwyd since 1974.* London: The Stationary Office.

Waterhouse, S. 2009. Issues and Experience (E mail Personal Communication, 14 October 2009).

Williams, J., LeFrancois, B. & Copperman, J. 2001. *Mental Health Services That Work for Women: Survey Findings.* Canterbury: Tizard Centre, University of Kent.

Williams, J. 2005. Women's mental health; taking inequality into account. *Social Perspectives in Mental Health.* Edited by J. Tew, London: Jessica Kingsley.

Chapter 7

The Assessment of Lesbian and Gay Prospective Foster Carers: Twenty Years of Practice and What has Changed?

Helen Cosis Brown

Introduction

This chapter draws on the findings of a small, explorative, qualitative study I undertook in the autumn of 2009; building on a colleague's and my own previous work addressing the content and quality of the assessments of lesbian and gay men prospective foster carers (Brown 1991, Brown and Cocker 2008, Cocker and Brown 2010). This chapter provides an overview of key changes to the legislative framework relevant to this area of social work practice and considers relevant findings from the Wakefield Inquiry (Parrott et al. 2007).

In the study I considered social work practitioners' ideas about the implications of changes in this area of social work practice and the impact they thought those changes had on the quality and content of their assessments of prospective lesbian and gay foster carers. I also examined if being located within a fostering agency that had experience of assessing lesbian and gay men as prospective foster carers affected the quality and the content of the assessment of lesbian and gay prospective foster carers, and if so how?

The research study, informing this chapter, consisted of two focus groups conducted with social workers in an Independent Fostering Agency (*n*=6) in the South East of England and one in a local authority fostering team (*n*=7) also in the South East of England. The focus groups were taped and the content of the tapes transcribed. These transcriptions were then read for themes that emerged from the discussions.

The local authority team was located in a London borough that had considerable experience of assessing lesbian and gay prospective adopters. Although the fostering team in this borough had less experience of assessing lesbian and gay prospective foster carers than their adoption colleagues, between all the team members they had accrued significant experience. One of the social workers within the local authority team had experience of the assessment of lesbian and gay foster carers going back to the early 1990s. The social workers, however, in the independent fostering agency team had no experience of assessing lesbian and gay foster carers. One of the independent fostering agency social work team members had been a member of a local authority fostering panel that had approved lesbian and gay applicants. She was therefore able to bring this experience to the discussion. This independent fostering agency team also had experience of working with two sets of foster carers who had undertaken introductions for their foster children to their new adoptive families; one being a lesbian couple and the other a gay male couple.

Despite the different levels of experience between the teams, one of the interesting findings from this small study was that the discussions within both teams were remarkably similar. One of the questions I wished to explore in undertaking these two focus groups was whether or not the experience of assessing lesbian and gay foster carers had an impact on the teams' thinking in this area of social work practice. The findings from this study indicated that the experience of undertaking assessments had little or no impact in differentiating the quality of the discussions between the local authority and the independent fostering agency teams. What was notable was the level of sophisticated discussion, confidence and critical thinking within both the teams. I have argued elsewhere that:

> in my experience capable social work practitioners work capably with all service
> users and carers and, similarly, incompetent ones work incompetently with all
> (Brown 2005:270).

What was notable was that both fostering teams had amassed considerable experience of assessment of a diverse group of prospective foster carers per se, and were confident assessing individuals and couples irrespective of their gender, sexuality, religion, ethnicity or single or couple status. For example, the independent fostering agency team had experience of assessing a transgender applicant as well as single male carers and although the issues may be different from those raised in the assessment of lesbians and gay men, these experiences had meant that they had had to think about a number of questions related to the quality and content of their assessments, particularly regarding sex, gender and sexuality.

Reviewing the past and considering the present

In the last five years there have been a number of publications reviewing the past as it relates to social work/social care with lesbians and gay men (Fish 2007, Brown 2008, Brown and Kershaw 2008, Fish 2009) and in particular lesbians and gay men and foster care (Hicks 2005, Brown and Cocker 2008). In preparing for writing this chapter I was struck by the number of similar papers. Indeed, the title I had chosen for this particular chapter was one that yet again looked backwards. Why, in 2010, are a number of academics taking this historical positioning whilst writing about social work/social care and lesbians and gay men; particularly as this 'looking back' is unusual for social work academics? My understanding of this interest in looking back is that quite simply, the rate of social and legislative change, relevant to lesbians and gay men, has been so considerable in the last twenty years that social work academics interested in this area are needing 'to take stock'. This seems to have been particularly the case since the passing of the Equality Act 2006 and its Section 81 related Sexual Orientation Regulations 2007. Fish argues that 'recent legislation marks a watershed in lesbian, gay and bisexual people's access to services...' (Fish 2007:221). It is this 'watershed' that we are trying to understand and consider what its impact is, and will be, on social work practice.

The legislative changes for lesbians and gay men as they pertain to social work that Fish refers to, have been considerable and are covered elsewhere (Fish 2007, Brown and Kershaw 2008). For the purposes of this chapter suffice it to say that in going from the legal position of twenty years ago to where we are now we have witnessed considerable legal and policy change. Twenty years ago the criminalization of some male same sex sexual activities, contributing to negative discrimination against gay men, was still on the statute books, and the persistent pursuit of lesbians and gay men by the British Conservative government from 1979, portraying them as the archetypal enemy of the family, was the norm. The period since 1997, with the election of the New Labour government, has seen the re-positioning of lesbians and gay men in the UK as a group that is legally protected from negative discrimination. This new position has come to fruition through both the repealing of discriminatory legislation and the passing of a number of new Acts including: the Adoption and Children Act 2002; the Civil Partnership Act 2004; the Equality Act 2006 and its related Sexual Orientation Regulations 2007 and the Equality Act 2010. These legal changes have not been won easily and some of the debates that have accompanied their passage through the House of Commons and the House of Lords bear witness to the fact that sometimes public opinion lags behind legal change.

Hicks (2005) provides us with a thorough coverage of the history of lesbian and gay fostering and adoption in the UK and links this to the changing legal and policy landscape. He looks, as well, at the development of lesbian and gay foster carers and adopters' organizations and lobbying groups such as the Lesbian and Gay Foster and Adoptive Parents Network, the Positive Parenting Campaign and Pink Parents UK. He also notes the national conferences organized by lesbians and gay men addressing adoption and fostering since 1988 and the impact such initiatives have had (Hicks 2005). The increasing visibility of lesbian and gay foster carers is set in the context of critical debates about the meaning of 'the family' and what its constituent parts should or could be. The critical analysis of 'the family' and social work's relationship to it has been part of social work thinking since the 1970s.

> The concept of the universality of the family is valid only in so far as account is taken of these diverse patterns, and when it is not used to force this diversity in to a uniform shape, or prove the intrinsic superiority of a particular form (Statham 1978:37). The diversity of family forms, their meanings, our understandings of

them and their relationship to the State are still contested (Weeks et al. 2001, Cahill and Tobias 2007).

During the early 1990s the Conservative government made several concerted efforts to limit the possibility of lesbians and gay men parenting either through: access to fertility services (the Embryology Act 1990), adopting (Department of Health 1992) or fostering (Department of Health 1990); in all cases their efforts failed. The Conservative Government's one success in this arena was the passing of Section 28 of the Local Government Act 1988. This section prevented local authorities using their resources in such a way that might be interpreted as 'promoting homosexuality' as well as forbidding 'promoting the teaching in any maintained school of homosexuality as a pretended family relationship'. Section 28 had little 'teeth' and indeed there were no successful prosecutions under it during its life time. However, it did have symbolic power in that it created anxiety within local authorities who might, as a result, have become more cautious in their pursuit of equality for lesbians and gay men. Section 28 was repealed in 2000 in Scotland and 2003 in England.

The speed of change regarding the legal position of lesbians and gay men, which has placed them on the same footing as their heterosexual counterparts, has been so fast that it can be argued it has outstripped the rate of change in public opinion. I have argued elsewhere that social workers are part of the public and some of those social workers might have found the speed of change too fast:

> Changing the law is one thing, changing social workers' attitudes is another. It appears that whilst there generally seems to be more tolerance and acceptance of lesbian and gay lifestyles there is no room for complacency, because … despite positive legislative changes, homophobic attitudes, prejudice and discrimination still exists. Legislation does not force people to change their views, however it does require them to be more tolerant and treat people alike.(Brown and Kershaw 2008:129).

This places social workers in the field of fostering in an interesting position. They are required by law to treat lesbian and gay applicants the same as their heterosexual applicants. However public opinion remains ambivalent towards lesbian and gay families. Both fostering and adoption have played a significant part in the creation of lesbian and gay families, despite some social workers reflecting society's ambivalence towards them (Hicks and McDermott 1999).

The Wakefield inquiry

An outcome of this ambivalence can be the creation of organizational and practitioner anxiety when working with lesbians and gay men. Some of this anxiety relates to negotiating unfamiliar territory. When working with groups which have been historically negatively discriminated against, social workers can feel anxious that they will be accused of also being negatively discriminatory. Another possible outcome can be the over focusing on the sexual orientation of the applicant/s in the assessment process or conversely the complete ignoring of the applicant/s sexuality:

> The Independent Inquiry into the Circumstances of Child Sexual Abuse by two Foster Carers in Wakefield – (Parrott et al. 2007) ... noted that the 'homosexuality' of the foster carers became the primary focus of social work anxiety. This happened at the expense of holistic considerations of both the carers' potential and their actual foster care practice. (Cocker and Brown 2010:20).

This important inquiry report recorded a number of problematic dynamics about how the gay male couple who were eventually imprisoned for sexually abusing looked-after children who were in their foster care were assessed, supervised and reviewed. The inquiry report in effect provides us with a case study of where matters related to the assessment of lesbian and gay foster carers went very wrong. It is important that we learn the lessons from this inquiry report. For my study, while preparing for conducting the focus groups with the local authority and independent fostering agency social workers, I noted a number of points from the report as I wanted to see if the social workers had taken on board the report's findings and how those findings might have influenced their foster care assessment practices.

In June 2006 two gay male foster carers who had been approved by Wakefield Council were given prison sentences for the sexual abuse of boys who had been fostered by them. The resulting inquiry report noted that the social workers demonstrated anxiety about being perceived as discriminatory, as well as demonstrating an inability to discriminate appropriately:

> [...] alongside anxieties on their part about being or being seen as prejudiced against gay people. The fear of being discriminatory led them to fail to discriminate between the appropriate and the abusive. Discrimination based on prejudice is not acceptable, especially not in social work or any public service. Discrimination founded on a professional judgement on a presenting issue, based on knowledge, assessed evidence and interpretation, is at the heart of good social work practice. These anxieties about discrimination have deep roots, we argue – in social work training, professional identity and organizational cultures... (Parrott et al. 2007:4).

Parrott et al also noted that: the assessment of the couple had

> 'failed to cover important psycho-social features of them as individuals and of their relationship with each other' (2007:38)

In addition they recorded that there had been a failure to address the problematic dynamics that built up between social workers as well as other professionals and the carers; and that there emerged an organizational position that developed towards these carers that new worrying information failed to influence. One of the informants to the Inquiry said:

> I think that one of the problems was that the family placement team were very clear that we've got these carers and they are unique ... the fact that they were a gay foster couple ... we need to do everything to support them, to help them remain foster carers really and that was very clearly coming across even though we were sort of saying, although not stating specifically that we felt the boys were being abused but were saying that we've got numerous concerns about these carers that need dealing with and ... whatever we were saying I felt was not really being listened to one hundred per cent because ultimately they wanted these foster carers to remain foster carers (2007:74).

Munro argues that practitioners should keep judgments under constant critical review and that they have to accept the possibility that their assessment might have been wrong (2008). In this Wakefield case it seems that this was an example of what Janis (1982) named 'Groupthink'. Janis is referring here to when a group or organization develop a perception of a situation which they then rigidly adhere to irrespective of information that might contradict that perception. The group's perception of a situation becomes to them a reality. The quote above denotes just such a phenomenon. Dissension from the organizational or Wakefield foster team's position regarding their view of these carers was not only difficult but also unlikely.

Findings from the LA and IFA focus groups

I met with both the independent fostering agency and local authority fostering teams which were located in the South East of England in the autumn of 2009. At the start of each of the focus groups I asked the individual members to complete a short questionnaire which asked for details of their ethnicity, age, gender, sexuality, years since qualification and years working in the field of foster care. Completion of this questionnaire was voluntary; two participants chose not complete it. In total I met with thirteen social workers. Of the thirteen, six described themselves as white British, three as Black British, one as Black African and one as Bangladeshi. Their ages ranged from between 20–30 to over 60. All of those who completed the forms described themselves as heterosexual. The total experience post qualification between them was 138 years and their cumulated time in foster care was 72 years. In terms of experience, the independent fostering agency were the most experienced in terms of time in social work post qualifying and also time spent in the field of fostering.

I asked both groups the same questions about what they perceived to be the same as well as different in the assessment of lesbians and gay men as compared to the assessment of heterosexual carers, and if they thought there had been changes in this area of practice in the last twenty years. I also asked them if and how the Wakefield inquiry had impacted on their assessment practices.

What was the same as well as different in the assessment of lesbians and gay men as compared to the assessment of heterosexual carers?

What should be the same and what should be different in the assessment of prospective foster carers has been a question within the literature since 1991. Both Brown (1991) and Hicks (2005) conclude that the assessment process and content need to be the same as well as different. Hicks, writing about the assessment of lesbian and gay foster carers, argues that:

> it is important to remember that assessing lesbians and gay men is not just 'the same' as assessing heterosexuals. There are areas particular to living as a gay or lesbian family in the UK that need consideration and discussion (Hicks 2005:52).

Writing fourteen years earlier I stated that:

> much of the debate about gay and lesbian parenting has centred on whether the assessment process should be the same for lesbian and gay applicants as it is for heterosexual applicants … the same thorough assessment should take place, but in addition the following areas should be addressed: the individual's experience of their homosexuality, their own and their family's response historically; how confident they feel in relation to their sexual orientation, how comfortable they are as lesbians or gay men; how homophobia and heterosexism have impinged on their lives and how they feel they've dealt with this, and what present coping devices they use; what are their present relationships – sexual, emotional, supportive, family, etc. How do they negotiate homophobia within close relationships, e.g. siblings; with reference to the future, how they have thought about relating to birth parents of foster children, how they have thought about relationships with outside carers, e.g. schools, playgroups, child minders. How much investigation have they done regarding attitudes of local institutions …. How they would help a child who experienced prejudice because of their carer's sexual orientation (Brown 1991:16).

The additional areas that I suggested should be explored in the assessment of lesbian and gay prospective foster carers were incorporated into the British Association for Adoption and Fostering good practice guidance on the recruiting, assessing and supporting of lesbian and gay carers and adopters (Mallon and Betts 2005).

The focus groups reflected this debate about whether the assessment of all carers should be the same or whether there should be some differences. What was interesting was that in both the independent fostering agency team as well as the local authority team this question was still open to debate. Both teams thought that considering this area made them more critical in their thinking about assessments being undertaken with heterosexual prospective carers. Susan from the independent fostering agency summed this up when talking about the assessment of lesbians and gay men's couple relationships, she said:

> I think I would be less inclined to make assumptions about the relationships …, I've more experience of heterosexual couples, whereas with same sex couples I think I'd be more careful to ask for the detail of their relationship. I hope I do that with heterosexual couples but I can see that it would be much easier to make assumptions.

Assia from the LA team reflecting on an initial visit she had undertaken with a lesbian couple who were applying to foster thought her assessments were the same irrespective of someone's sexual orientation:

> I ask the same questions I ask heterosexual couples in the initial visit, ask them about their relationship, ask them about how long they've been together, how they would work together as a couple, their motivations and because they're not going to have children of their own what was motivating them to foster which would be the same question I would ask a heterosexual couple who is childless. I felt I did the same thing, I would ask the same questions.

Gloria from the local authority team noted some areas of difference that she felt were important:

> I think the other thing that can be different is about the need to have a discussion about some of the discrimination they're going to meet when they start fostering from within the community and how we're going to help them but also how resilient they are about actually being able to manage that as well, because if they're not resilient, you know, it's not going to work.

The need for resilience was a theme that emerged within both focus group discussions. The resilience that they were looking for was evident in a local authority's initial assessment of a lesbian couple which Delia described:

> I asked them what their relationship was like with other people around the local community just to get a grasp on how they were dealing with being discriminated against. But speaking to the couple it was eye-opening for me because where they were living they had very good friends and they said yes they had been discriminated against or felt that people were looking at them in a funny way but because of their confidence, they were confident about their relationship, they were very secure, other people didn't find it very easy to point fingers at them. Which meant because they were secure in their own relationship any foster

child coming into their home would feel that sense of security. So that's a very positive thing.

This discussion about the need for resilience raised the question in the independent fostering agency team about whether or not we are asking more of gay and lesbian foster care applicants than we do of heterosexual ones. This was best articulated in a discussion which took place primarily between Janet and Albert:

Janet – So are you saying that you think they would need special qualities over and above those that you would expect of heterosexuals?

Albert – Maybe, yeah.

Janet – But I don't know whether we should be or why you might be....

Albert – I'm saying that lesbian and gay carers are going to potentially come across situations that are difficult and therefore they are going to need emotional resources to deal with that.

Janet – But all foster carers are going to come across difficult situations. I'm not sure that we would want different qualities .... Can they do the job is what you're asking, whether it be of a single carer, a heterosexual couple, a gay couple ... each situation will throw up particular potential difficulties that you need to identify and explore ....

One of the areas that Hicks and McDermott identified in their research looking at the experience of lesbians and gay men being assessed as foster carers and adopters was 'that many talked about the gender concerns raised by social workers and /or panels' (1999:162) . This was particularly related to domestic arrangements and the question of who does what within the home and within the community. The assumption being that within heterosexual families' roles and responsibilities are usually divided according to gender (Brown 1992, Weeks et al. 2001). This concern emerged within the focus groups: Keisha from the independent fostering agency thinking about what would be the same and what would be different in the assessment of lesbians and gay men said:

I suppose in terms of what would I do the same; to look at how they are with their own family, how they are connected to the community and how they are settled as a couple, you know it's all the same things that I would look at. Say if it was two men in a partnership you might think well if they didn't have any children themselves you might think well its always the lady in the man-wife situation who goes to the school and makes contact with the school, you know you make these assumptions but then you think well if its two men in a partnership, who would take on that role? What is their experience in that role? So you'd kind of be thinking how do they see themselves within the community?

This led on to a discussion about the very different domestic arrangements that all couples have and the need to not make assumptions about any couple but rather, in the words of Chantelle from the independent fostering agency:

I feel fine trying to pull it apart and saying OK let's scrap the initial model and look at what happens in your family. With a heterosexual couple there is a danger that we can make generalized assumptions.

Both the local authority and the independent fostering agency teams were committed to detailed and rigorous assessments of all applicants irrespective of their sexual orientation. Included in this rigorous approach was critical analysis of the quality of the relationship between the assessor and the applicants. Chantelle from the independent fostering agency summed this up when she looked back at an assessment where the sexuality of one of the applicants had needed to be fully explored:

What you're looking for in any assessment is people getting why your, understanding why you're asking the question, you might have to explain why you're asking the question, that's fair enough but kind of tuning into that and being able to show insight and openness in exploring that theme with you. You'd want them to understand why you were exploring how that might be for a child. The problem in that particular assessment was that it was kind of like drawing teeth at the beginning and that it's a kind of hidden subject and at some stages there was a very limited understanding as to why I was asking the questions.

The LA team was aware that some lesbian and gay men are wary of how they might be treated in the assessment process because of past experience of negative discrimination and that this can have an impact on the quality of the relationship that they establish with the assessor. Amina voiced a concern as follows:

I think I'd be wary of people's increased sensitivity really and expecting to be discriminated against and the initial, maybe first half an hour, is about getting over that barrier and thinking of ways of working together positivity. That's been my experience on occasions. They've been, I think, very surprised about how welcoming we are but still have been a little bit apprehensive about … I suppose things like, – 'we'll need to speak to family members' – if there's been some rift associated with their sexuality and disclosure and us having to be clear about why we have to undertake those interviews.

Another local authority team member Ola talked about how her experiences as a black woman helped her make links with lesbians and gay men's experiences of discrimination and how this, in her experience, helped the working relationship during the assessment:

When I did my assessment it was about their resilience and how they coped with telling friends and family about their sexuality and how people also responded to that. But I think I based some aspects of my assessment on my sense of being a black woman with regard to different types of racism and discrimination I've experienced. I linked it to their experience of their sexuality and I think I worked it like that and it worked quite easy for me and I felt quite comfortable about it as well so I think that's how I turned the assessment around.

Assia from the local authority team having summed up what she was looking for in carers, which included having the skills and knowledge to undertake the 'fostering task that has become increasingly complex' said that she consciously considered:

Whether we can work with people, how has the dialogue been between us and have we been able to establish that professional understanding.

Has this area of practice changed in the last twenty years and if so how?

Hicks noted the considerable degree of change that there has been in this field since 1988:

There are now greater numbers of lesbians and gay men applying, gaining approval and having children placed in their care, although this tends to be concentrated in certain inner city or progressive authorities (2005:52).

He also records the increasing confidence of applicants who are open from the start about their sexuality. The findings from the focus groups in my study reflect a general increase in confidence on behalf of the social work assessors. This increase in confidence means that both assessors and applicants can potentially be more open, clear and challenging in their assessments. Gloria, from the local authority team, said that she was aware of this need for confidence:

Thinking back to an assessment I did, now this was back in the 90s, I think I approached it exactly the same way I would as if it was a single heterosexual woman, as I would have done any other assessment. But I think actually what I learnt from that was this bit about people being resilient and positive and this particular person wasn't in retrospect very secure in her own identity as a lesbian woman. When we started to place children with her they very very quickly homed in on that and really really quickly picked that up and actually became very abusive and because she wasn't secure she wasn't able to deal with that. I think we learnt a lot from that assessment about the need for people to be very secure about themselves which is no different from other people really.

A more appropriately intrusive and challenging assessment of this foster carer might have revealed more about her lack of confidence and insecurity.

Chantelle from the independent fostering agency noted real changes in the placement of children with approved lesbian and gay foster carers when she thought back to her previous foster panel experience:

> The panel I was on only had the one experience of each gender but the male carers were assessed and approved with no problem but they were never ever ever used in my lifetime in that job. So the politically correct thing was to put on your strap line 'you can be black, white, young, old, gay, straight', but there's other ways to dodging the problem, which was that they never had children placed with them for whatever reason. That in itself raises other sort of questions. Just because you can be assessed as being able to do the job and get through that assessment process with whoever it is that approves you doesn't mean that someone else is going to agree and then use you as a foster carer.

Gloria in the local authority team made a similar point as that raised by Chantelle as follows:

> When I worked in fostering in the 90s there was a very ambivalent attitude about whether or not we wanted to recruit gay or lesbian foster carers. On the one hand there was this message of 'yes recruit' but then there was also another message that was coming from the Authority about 'oh God we're going to get headlines in the papers about recruiting gay and lesbian foster carers' we're going to get loads of negative publicity. I think actually we've moved on from that, I don't think that that's there anymore. I think that we now genuinely welcome people.

This local authority team went on to talk about their pro-active recruitment of lesbians and gay men, advertising in the gay press and the local authority fostering team providing information sessions at the lesbian and gay London Pride festival.

Assia, from the same team, noted the following changing attitudes of social workers about placing children with lesbian and gay carers:

> I think we have learnt quite a lot on an individual level as well as on a professional level when we think about the assessment of lesbians and gay men as foster carers because I remember when I was in my previous team in child protection there was a same sex couple from an agency. One of my colleagues wanted to place children with that couple and it was a big issue for, not necessarily for the team, but particularly pressure was coming from various other teams, as well as from the child and their family and the Guardian who was involved. I think probably .... I think in general we have moved on. We have done quite a lot and our approach and our attitude has changed in a positive way.

The independent fostering agency team had experience of working with heterosexual foster carers who were undertaking introductory work for foster children they were caring for where the new permanent family was gay. Janet noted changes in this area of practice:

> My sense is that gay and lesbian foster carers and adopters have been well and truly established as in the mainstream in many London local authorities. So we're talking about children, and these were two bright baby girls, who would be plum children for adoption. Two of them! Two little girls; two children to die for. Now five years ago if you were gay or lesbian you would have taken the leftovers in terms of children for adoption, you would never have been offered the sort of child that people would be willing to fight for.

One of the dynamics that the Wakefield Inquiry (Parrott et al. 2007) noted was a degree of fearfulness on the part of the social worker, when assessing and working with lesbians and gay men, about being considered negatively discriminatory. This 'fear' was not evident in either of these teams. This might have been different in the past. They were aware of this potential dynamic and the Inquiry Report had emphasized this for them. Susan from the independent fostering agency said:

> It makes all of us sort of think because we are doing assessments with a variety of people, we have to address all issues. It showed me we can't sort of back away from tackling issues because of our insecurities or for fear or being labelled as discriminatory so I think in that way its helpful to keep that in mind when you're undertaking any assessment.

Gloria from the local authority also said:

> I think the change is that we are more confident about lesbian and gay assessments. What I mean by that is that we are more confident about addressing the issues in the same way we would with any other carer. We're not worried about being told we're discriminating. We're confident about explaining why we're asking questions.

What was evident through the focus group discussions was that many of the recommendations of the Inquiry Report (Parrott et al. 2007) for both these teams were already in place. However, they had considered the Report's findings and for both teams they were reminded of the need for rigorous, thorough and analytical assessment of all aspects of applicants' lives irrespective of their sexuality. Albert, a member of the independent fostering agency team, was considering his work in a new light as a result of the Wakefield Inquiry report. He was working with a heterosexual couple where the detail of their relationship was gradually unfolding:

I'm referring to the couple who are taking time out from having children placed with them, who I met last week, the heterosexual couple. I think the whole Wakefield thing and talking about the psycho-social is so important. For that heterosexual couple really understanding the absolute importance of their relationship and how they are relating to each other and how that will have an effect on fostering, really breaking it down has been essential. I still see issues there and I think the sexuality and the relationship is absolutely critical in understanding and appreciating how those foster carers relate to each other and in turn relate to children.

Keisha, from the independent fostering agency team, summed up when she talked about some of the benefits of assessing lesbians and gay men as foster carers:

So what you're looking for is resilience and the ability to deal with either the specific questions that their history brings to the fore or whatever other problems fostering might throw at them. Because in a way with a gay couple, I think, it makes it easier to find issues that they may have had to deal with in their lives that you can talk about and relate to fostering and looked after children. Whereas sometimes Mr and Mrs Conventional you struggle to find anything in their lives that's been problematic that you can use to actually help them to get them to talk about how that might relate to fostering.

Summing up

Lesbians and gay men have experienced a period of unprecedented change in their social and legal position in the UK over the last twenty years. Those changes have been reflected in them being able to apply to be foster carers and where appropriate for them to be approved as foster carers. This small study showed that both the independent fostering agency and the local authority teams were aware of significant change in this area of practice. There were no obvious differences between the independent fostering agency and the local authority teams in what they discussed. Despite the varying levels of experience of assessing lesbians and gay men as prospective foster carers, this didn't seem to impact on the quality or content of the discussion. This might be to do with the geographical location of the teams and the fact that both teams are located in areas that have diverse communities including significant gay and lesbian populations.

Both teams were thoughtful and reflective in the discussion about the practice detail of their assessments and both were focused on the paramountcy of the child. Both were relatively confident and were not overly concerned about being accused of being negatively discriminatory. Both teams, through focusing on the assessment of lesbian and gay prospective foster carers, had considered the quality and the rigour of their assessment of heterosexual prospective foster carers, particularly regarding gender, domestic arrangements and sexuality. In addition the fostering teams saw resilience as being a key attribute that all potential foster carers needed. Overall the content of the discussions was quite different from the findings of the Wakefield Inquiry. However, retrospective discussions about practice that this study relied upon are not necessarily accurate indicators as to how people actually behave in the present or might behave in the future.

The social work practitioners in this study, when assessing lesbian and gay prospective foster carers, covered areas that they would address with all prospective foster carers, as well as those identified by Brown (1991) and Brown and Cocker (2008). The main change that can be noted from this research was the growth in confidence of social workers in undertaking this work.

References

Brown, H.C. 1991. Competent child-focused practice: Working with lesbian and gay carers. *Adoption and Fostering*. 15(2), 11–17.

Brown, H.C. 1992. Gender, sex and sexuality in the assessment of prospective carers. *Adoption and Fostering*, 16(2), 30–34.

Brown, H.C. and Kershaw, S. 2008. The legal context of working with lesbians and gay men. *Social Work Education*, 27(2),122–130.

Brown, H.C. 2008. Social work and sexuality, working with lesbians and gay men: What Remains the same and what is fifferent. *Practice: Social Work in Action*, 20(4), 265–276.

Brown, H.C. and Cocker, C. 2008. Lesbian and gay fostering and adoption: Out of the closet into the mainstream. *Adoption and Fostering*, 32(4), 19–30.

Cahill, S. & Tobias, S. 2007. *Policy Issues Affecting Lesbian, Gay, Bisexual, and Transgender Families,* Michigan: The University of Michigan Press.

Cocker, C. & Brown, H.C. 2010 Sex, Sexuality and Relationships: Developing Confidence and Discernment when Assessing Lesbian and Gay Prospective Adopters. *Adoption and Fostering*, 34(1), 20–32.

Department of Health 1990. *Foster placement (Guidance and Regulations)* consultation paper No 16, London: HMSO.

Department of Health and Welsh Office 1992. *Review of Adoption Law: Report to Ministers of an Interdepartmental Working Group*. Consultation document, London: HMSO.

Fish, J. 2007. Getting equal: the implications of new regulations to prohibit sexual orientation discrimination for health and social care. *Diversity in Health and Social Care*, 4(3), 221–228.

Fish, J. 2009. Invisible no more? Including, gay and bisexual people in social work and social care'. *Practice: Social Work in Action*, 21(1), 47–64.

Janis, I. 1982. Groupthink: psychological studies of policy decisions and fiascos, in *Effective Child Protection*, edited by E. Munro. London: The Stationary Office.

Hicks, S. 2005. Lesbian and gay foster care and adoption: A brief UK history. *Adoption and Fostering*, 29(3), 42–56.

Hicks, S. & McDermott, J. 1999. (Editors) *Lesbian and Gay Fostering and Adoption: Extraordinary yet Ordinary.* London: Jessica Kingsley Publishers.

Mallon, G.P. & Betts, B. 2005. *Recruiting, Assessing and Supporting Lesbian and Gay Carers and Adopters.* London: British Agency for Adoption and Fostering.

Munro, E. 2000. Improving reasoning in supervision. *Social Work Now*, 40, 3–10.

Parrott, B., MacIver, A. & Thoburn, J. 2007. *Independent Inquiry into the Circumstances of Child Sexual Abuse by Two Foster Carers in Wakefield.* Wakefield: Wakefield County Council.

Statham, D. 1978. *Radicals in Social Work.* London: Routledge and Kegan Paul.

Weeks, J., Heaphy, B. & Donovan, C. 2001. *Same Sex Intimacies: Families of Choice and Other Life Experiments.* London: Routledge.

Chapter 8

What is Personal? Reflecting on Heterosexuality

Joy Trotter

Introduction

Sexuality and sexual identity are neglected dimensions in social work. Though social work literature has begun to unravel some of the complexities involved in this area of human experience, differing epistemologies have resulted in a plethora of approaches. In this chapter I argue that feminist literature helps to decipher broader meanings of sexuality and enables a re-orientation of the sexual self with the personal realm of experience. Using three key areas identified as meaningful in feminist scholarship, I trace the notion of sexuality, and in particular, heterosexuality through three dimensions: emotions, relationships and identity. I conclude the chapter with a personal reflection which draws from the feminist notion that personal experience is a relevant and valid form of knowledge.

Social work has always been interested in the more personal and private aspects of life and has scrutinized, adjudicated and reflected on these from a range of perspectives and with a variety of motives. It has also been argued for some time that elements of self-awareness, unconscious processes and the more private and personal aspects of our lives are crucial to a wide range of research and practice settings and professional abilities. However, although much of what is deemed to be private and personal relates to our sexuality, this often seems to be overlooked. In social work, when sexuality is acknowledged, it is often either over-scrutinized if considered 'deviant' (and especially if related to service-users), or over-looked if considered 'normal' (and especially if it relates to ourselves).

The chapter will begin with a discussion of three main strands of what social work means by personal – emotions, relationships and identities – and in relating these to gender and sexualities, will explore how heterosexuality is differently portrayed and understood in a range of social work and other literature. It will then also consider a number of recently published policy documents and practice guidelines and, alongside the *Code of Ethics for Social Work*, will argue that requirements and expectations for practice are conflicting and compromising in relation to gender and sexuality. In conclusion, using illustrations from personal experience, the chapter will end by suggesting that many of the difficulties are linked to heterosexuality and that: a) social work research and education needs to revisit feminist understandings of heterosexuality; b) documents relating to conduct and governance should be re-written in order that they might more honestly account for the realities of heterosexual life; and c) heterosexual women and men might offer some solutions by being more truthful about personal issues in their professional practice.

The chapter probably began many years ago when I started reading and thinking about my own sexuality as heterosexual. Many books have inspired me since then, but two have more recently made a considerable impact – for very different reasons. The first, a novel set in very recent times, is a vivid and intense account of young people's heterosexual relationships over one summer in Middlesbrough in the North East of England (Milward 2008). It has reminded me of my own youthful haphazard and often hazardous sexual experiences and encounters in the 1960s when many young women's lives were (and seem still to be) boring and terrifying in equal measures. It made me question how these experiences might have affected my work (and especially my relationships) in social work practice and education over the years. The second book is an academic text which focuses on heterosexuality and families (Hockey, Meah and Robinson 2007). This book asks what it means to be heterosexual, how implicit meanings about heterosexuality are communicated between generations and what young people think when they anticipate adult heterosexuality. The authors provide a detailed and enlightening account of their research which, using a life history approach, interviewed 72 men and women in East Yorkshire within 20 extended families and across three generations. Their research exposes a rich seam of diversity with private narratives and 'unruly emotions' (181). The authors suggest that not only does heterosexuality 'transcend' sexual matters, it also influences gender identities and life events – both mundane and significant. In conclusion the authors wonder whether 'sex' has anything to do with heterosexuality, rather suggesting that:

> [...] the mundanity of oppressive heterosexual relationships contributes to the power and inequality which characterizes them; yet in addition, can encompass the embodied, materially grounded moments which signal profound transitions, both into and out of such relationships. (Hockey, Meah and Robinson 2007: 188).

Following on from ideas like Kitzinger's (2005), who showed how the unrelenting and assumed heteronormative social order is maintained in mundane social interactions, Hockey and her colleagues offer a dual approach of 'mundane' and 'extreme' to understand the complexity and diversity of heterosexual experiences. Troubles and secrets featured regularly:

> Many interviewees explored with us those aspects of their heterosexual lives which troubled them. Yet despite this openness, for some their troubles were felt to be so stigmatizing that these were precisely the areas omitted from their accounts (115). [...] secrecy prevailed ... and indeed masked transgressive

heterosexuality among members of all three generations. (Hockey, Meah and Robinson 2007:122).

What are these troubles and secrets and how do they affect us in our lives and our work? Are the romantic ideas about love or the unproblematized notions about monogamy in heterosexual relations clouding our judgements? Are our 'family practices' (which, according to Hockey and her colleagues, are a set of understandings which reflect social identities, proscribe particular behaviours and construe meanings about sexuality, gender, respectability and social class), influencing our professional practice? Are our own experiences of desire and disappointment, passion and pain, crucial elements of who we are and how we relate to others, or just incidental bits of our personal histories? What is personal? Why don't we know?

As social workers we are faced with difficult issues on a daily basis, many relating to sexuality, for example rape and sexual violence, disease, disability and infertility, child sexual abuse, sex trafficking and pornography. Many of these are present in our own lives too and, as this is rarely acknowledged, it is hard to guess how many of us are involved and affected personally. Sometimes the line between what is personal and what is work is less than clear (Charles 1993, Leech and Trotter 2006, Myers 2008, Shernoff 2004) and many personal experiences are of relevance to professional ethics and social work values (Freel 2003, Goodchild 2007, O'Connell Davidson 1995). It has recently been argued that social work needs to pay greater attention to the understanding of and teaching about 'everyday sexuality' (Christie 2006, Dunk 2007, Hicks 2008) and some have begun to suggest new ways of thinking about social practices and categories and the production of sexual meanings in our work. These ideas need to be explored further and must address heterosexuality and gender more centrally and routinely than has been done so far.

A look at some of the literature

As suggested earlier, social workers have always operated in areas where personal and private issues and relationships are at the heart of their work, and have investigated, assessed and reflected on these in different ways and with differing motives (for example, Biestek 1989, Hugman 2009, Morrison 2007, Pugh 2007). They have also drawn on and been influenced by the literature of other disciplines in these areas, and this continues in the twenty-first century. However, social work's willingness or ability to learn from and assimilate others' ideas about gender and sexuality have been rather haphazard. Although there was a great deal about gender in social work in the 1980s, and a growing literature base in sociology and psychology about sexuality, it wasn't until the mid-1990s that academic papers and social work texts addressed social work and sexuality (Bremner and Hillin 1994, Cosis Brown 1998, Logan and Kershaw 1994).

Most of these earlier texts, however, only focused on lesbian and gay sexualities. More recently it has been argued that lesbian, gay, bisexual and transgender (LGBT) sexualities are no longer invisible in health and social care (Fish 2009), but heterosexuality is still 'not there' as a visible and acknowledged identity. Until heterosexuality is acknowledged, it is not available for scrutiny, and not truly assessable. Its problems remain hidden, silenced, ignored. Lesbian and gay social workers and service users have recognized for some time that social work has seemed reluctant to admit its connections with sexuality policies, or to address sexuality issues in education or practice (Trotter, Kershaw and Knott 2008). This reluctance may in some way be linked to the continuing invisibility of heterosexuality and its associated problems. There continues to be, however, a large body of work relating to emotions, relationships and identities in social work and social care, but how much of this addresses gender and sexuality, let alone heterosexuality, is debatable.

Emotions

Sociology and psychology have considered adults' emotions in some depth (Smart 2007, Burman 2009) and have debated the benefits and dangers of emotional intelligence and literacy, the importance of positive as well as negative emotions, and even the existence of love in our social negotiations and relationships. Others have also begun to acknowledge the often emotional nature of research (Dickson-Swift et al. 2009, Hayes and Campbell 2005) and education (Moon 2004, Ryan 2001) and the importance of recognizing feelings. Interestingly, in youth work, Collander-Brown (2005) says workers rarely use or speak about their own feelings (though they are 'put to use' indirectly – 44), because the focus is on young people's feelings which are already 'complex enough … introducing the worker's feelings would make the task almost impossible' (44).

Social work literature also addresses emotions. It often prescribes how workers should feel about their clients (empathy, acceptance, and so on) but, as Shaw (2008) points out, it does not always tell us how to achieve these emotions 'in a pressured, frustrating and sometimes frightening environment' (Shaw 2008:24). The acknowledgement and management of strong emotions such as anger, frustration, fear and sorrow, continue to be researched and written about (Cooper and Lousada 2005) and require strategies for working with conflict, often without consent or collaboration (Ferguson 2005). However these rarely acknowledge, let alone address, sexualities (Fenge and Fannin 2009) and almost never allude to feelings of repugnance, desire, or other (positive or negative) sexual feelings (Fraser 2005, Hicks 2008, Plummer 2001).

Some authors do write about feelings around sexuality in the context of sexual assault and sexual safety. For example Barlow and Hall (2007) discuss the management of students' feelings whilst on placement and give examples of women students encountering sexual offenders, where one (who had been 'sexually assaulted as a teenager') was 'flooded with unresolved feelings' (403) and another felt 'extreme discomfort' when she encountered sexual harassment from prisoners at an adult detention centre (405). The emotional context of learning in social work has also been addressed (Trotter 2006a) and there are texts which are directed at social work students (Knott and Scragg 2007) about emotions. Butler (2007) emphasizes the need for social workers to be able to reflect on their own and their clients' emotions, arguing that it is an integral part of our practice. She is astonished to note that emotions are not referred to in the National Occupational Standards (NOS), the Subject Benchmark statement, nor in the General Social Care Council's Code of Conduct. Smethurst (2007) is similarly surprised to find that emotions are not referred to in Key Roles or standards for post-qualifying training, and points out that this is despite the fact that 'social workers often engage with particularly distressing and emotionally challenging situations' (Smethurst 2007:99). Wallis (2007) clearly demonstrates how the neglect of emotions is commonplace and understandable in practice, but can be disastrous in child protection work.

However, most of this literature refers to negative emotions – fear, shock, horror, hostility, aggression, distaste, intimidation, anxiety, abandonment, loss, relief, disgust, envy, shame. Very few refer to positive emotions and none to sexual feelings or desires.

Relationships

Our relationships have also been explored from a range of perspectives, including our associations with clients, research subjects, students, colleagues and our own personal relationships (Cant 2006; Mackinnon 2004; Morris 1997; Swanberg and Macke 2006). Elements of risk around sexuality in these relationships have been greatly scrutinized in recent years, especially the potential difficulties around sexual safety regarding clients (Green, Butt and King 2002, Karban 2007, Stevens et al. 2008, Yacoub and Hall 2007). This work has focused on both risks to us *from* clients, and risks *to* clients (from ourselves). Other aspects of our relationships with clients have also been addressed. In work with young people for example, the relationship between the worker and the young person may be the central and most important factor (Collander-Brown 2005, Ruch 2005). Balen and Crawshaw (2006) point to an array of contentious and difficult relationships regarding sexuality and fertility issues in health settings. Cull (2006) refers to young people with Congenital Adrenal Hyperplasia (CAH) and other similar conditions, and highlights the lack of communication throughout their childhoods and adolescence with any adult, despite having so much to communicate about sexual matters. Similarly, Cincotta, Childs and Eichenfield (2006) discuss sexuality in relation to growing up HIV-Positive when professionals are reluctant to communicate. As discussed elsewhere (Leech and Trotter 2005), social workers' reticence, particularly in communicating about sexuality with young lesbian and gay people, might be linked to their own memories which they elude by avoiding talking about or even raising the issues of sexuality with their young clients.

Relationships with research subjects (Coffey 2002) and with students (Carter and Jeffs 1995) have been less thoroughly examined in terms of sexuality, but our relationships with each other as colleagues have almost been entirely overlooked. A recent issue of one professional magazine included a piece about child protection mistakes being linked to managerial style which is described as 'sterile' and staff relationships which are described as 'controlling', 'overbearing' and even 'bullying' (Brand 2009:10). However, given that much of child abuse involves *sexual* abuse, it is paradoxical that issues of sexuality are not alluded to.

Similarly overlooked in the literature is any allusion to our own personal relationships with family members, partners and friends. Many, if not most of these relationships are hugely important to us, many are a source of support and joy, some are otherwise. Most of them have at least an element of sexuality in their history (for parents and children for example), if not in their current arrangements. However, although our personal relationships may be mentioned and even celebrated at work, they are in a social context and are not related to professional issues or competencies. Furthermore, the sexual elements of these personal relationships are overlooked and even denied, especially if they are problematic. For example, as many social workers are women, many will experience domestic violence or sexual aggression. How are these experiences expressed (or not) and how do they affect our relationships at work? Research from the United States suggests that the impact on work can be great (Swanberg and Macke 2006). According to Hirst and Cox (1996), 'our own life experiences reinforce our theoretical and personal understandings of "patriarchal relations"' (Hirst and Cox 1996:33) and therefore how we are and how we communicate to others.

According to Kirkman and her colleagues (2005), communication is a key factor in relationships, particularly when trying to talk about sex and sexuality. According to their research, mothers send mixed messages to their young daughters about their willingness to answer questions about sexual matters. This complicated process is referred to as being 'open with your mouth shut' (Kirkman et al. 2005) and demonstrates that a great deal of information is communicated without (sometimes despite) words, in our relationships with others, and much of the crucial information is not communicated at all. Not unlike the mothers in Kirkman and her colleagues' research, many liberal-minded social workers imply their willingness to embrace diversity around sexualities and to address sexual matters in their work; yet, reality often seems very different. Indeed, being liberal and fair-minded, even when reasonably well-informed and aware, does not seem to increase the amount of frank discussions about personal relationships or involvement in sexuality-related work (Trotter 2001). Most social workers continue to present a guarded and limited version of heterosexuality in their relationships:

> [...] constrained heterosexuality and virtual asexuality [are] adopted by many professionals in formal and informal structures around work. (Trotter 2006b: 299).

Perhaps it is felt that social and professional relationships between heterosexual social workers are only acceptable, or unthreatening, when they are inhibited, insipid and hiding all problems.

Identities

Whilst social workers are used to discussing and assessing emotions and relationships, they are often less familiar with notions of identity and may be less inclined to look for the literature relating to identities. According to Reynolds (2008), identity is 'a negotiated performance that may be performed differently for different sets of circumstances' and goes on to suggest that this is fashioned by the 'cultural resources', personal history and 'conversational turns' of the moment (Reynolds 2008:25). Who we are, and who we are perceived to be, is a crucial element of our professional persona and practice. Social workers have many identities, as well as their professional one. There are those associated with family such as carers, fathers, grandmothers or 'WAGS', and those linked to interests and associations like musicians, athletes and 'goths'. Our appearances also influence, if not determine our identity, for example our race, physicality, wearing a uniform, pregnancy.

The effect of our appearance on others has been much researched and debated, particularly in psychology (for example, Marlowe, Schneider and Nelson 1996, Raudenbush and Zellner 1997, Hargreaves and Tiggemann 2006), and often in relation to gender and discrimination (Frith and Gleeson 2004, Keery et al. 2005, Zaidel, Aarde and Baig 2005). However, although there have been explicit attempts to address appearance in relation to lesbian and gay sexualities (for example, National Lesbian and Gay Survey 1992, Winn and Nutt 2001), little has been established in relation to heterosexuality and appearance, and this has not been addressed in the social work literature.

Social workers whose sexualities are lesbian or gay may well be more practised at managing their identities at work. Satterly (2004), as a gay male therapist, suggests that carefully considered and well-prepared self-disclosure is a useful way to manage identities in practice using a matrix of 'reflective lenses'. However, many still feel the necessity to hide their sexuality because of vulnerabilities to homophobic abuse and prejudice (Carabine 2004, Trotter et al. 2009).

Other aspects of sexual identity have been discussed in health (Cant 2006), mental health (Ault and Brzuzy 2009), education (Paechter 2007) and social policy (Shildrick 2004), all of particular relevance to social work. In social work, a number of authors have considered identity relating to men as social workers (Hearn and Pringle 2006, Hicks 2001), and Scourfield (2003) shows that British social workers often represent their male colleagues in such ways as to distance them from their men clients, whom they regard as a 'threat', 'no use', irrelevant' and 'absent' (Scourfield 2003:89–100). Christie's (2006) research suggests that men social workers are often regarded as 'more able than 'ordinary men' to talk about personal and intimate aspects of life' and even the 'sexist' ones maybe less sexist than ordinary men (404) but, on the whole, 'men social workers are represented as either compensating for "absent fathers" and/ or representing potential risks to children and women' (Christie 2006:32).

There seems to be no parallel literature at all about women social workers' identities. Although a number of important texts have focused on gender (Orme 2001, Lyons and Taylor 2004, Scourfield 2003), gender issues (Dominelli 2002, Harding and Hamilton, 2009, Mullender 2002) and feminist perspectives in social work (Cox, Kershaw and Trotter 2000, White 2006), only few of them address sexuality and none consider heterosexuality in relation to women social workers. How do we women in social work portray our heterosexuality and how is it perceived by others? If it is true that we still cling to romantic ideas about love and unproblematized notions about monogamous heterosexuality, how do we manage our own (and our partners') infidelities and abuses? Indeed, are most of us heterosexual and in relationships with men (and children)? Does an alternative personal identity for women social workers pose any problems to clients, colleagues or employing organizations? Reynolds' (2008) research about 'troublesome' interactions around being single, may have particular relevance for social work as 'aloneness' is often construed as some sort of deficit or failure in our assessments of clients.

Part of the everyday routine for single women involves negotiating their way through and past category sets in which they either have no place, or need to explain in what ways they belong (Reynolds 2008:146–7).

Do these difficulties pertain to single women social workers too? What seems to have emerged from this glimpse at the literature is that little consideration is given to sexuality and sexual identities in social work, particularly in relation to heterosexuality and social workers themselves (especially women). Furthermore, despite the plethora of research data, academic papers and educative texts relating to all three elements of what I am considering as 'personal' (emotions, relationships and identities) in social work, and even an emerging body of work addressing lesbian and gay sexuality, most of this focuses on clients or on our experiences with clients; almost none relates to heterosexuality in any critical or scholarly way.

Documents about conduct and governance

Clearly much of the literature, both social work's and others', seems patchy and inconclusive about gendered relationships in the workplace, about the links between personal/private lives and professional lives, and about problems with heterosexuality. How do we know how we should proceed, particularly as we begin to address some of the important issues that have been raised in the literature? Perhaps the regulations and systems of governance offer some guidance.

In 2004 the General Social Care Council (GSCC) introduced a Code of Practice for English social care workers and their employers (GSCC 2004) which requires, amongst many things, that practitioners must 'strive to establish and maintain the trust and confidence of service users and carers' (Code 2) and inform employers 'where the practice of colleagues may be unsafe or adversely affecting standards of care' (Code 3.2). Furthermore, the code forbids forming 'inappropriate personal relationships with service users' (Code 5.4).

As part of its responsibilities for regulating the social care workforce in England, the GSCC maintains a register of staff and recently published information about conduct hearings (held as a result of their receiving information about social workers who may have breached the Codes of Practice). Their own newsletter (GSCC 2009a) reported that there had been over 55 hearings into the conduct of social workers and student social workers covering a whole range of allegations, from inappropriate personal relationships with service users to dishonesty on applications. As a result of these hearings, 25 people had been removed from the register, 8 suspended and 20 admonished. They also reported that a number of cases brought before the hearings had found periods of sustained and deliberate access to internet sites showing sexually explicit material using work equipment. Their statistics also showed that inappropriate relationships accounted for 40 per cent of conduct cases.

Interestingly, although the GSCC recently produced some analyses of gender, ethnicity and disability in relation to their registered social workers (GSCC 2009b), showing over 76% of them to be women, they do not appear to have analysed (or if they have, they have not shared the results) the gender of the 56 people removed, suspended or admonished, nor the 40% found to have had 'inappropriate relationships'. Their analyses made no mention of sexuality (GSCC 2009a). Were most of them heterosexual men?

Another organization which may influence the conduct of social workers is the British Association of Social Workers (BASW), which outlines the duties and responsibilities of the profession in a Code of Ethics for Social Work (BASW 2006). The code, which is actually a list of 'Values' which social work 'is committed to', state that social workers have a duty 'to ensure that their private conduct does not compromise the fulfilment of professional responsibilities, and to avoid behaviour which contravenes professional principles and standards or which damages the profession's integrity' (Value 3.4.2) and include two (out of six) sub-categories relating specifically to sexual behaviour:

- Not to engage in any form of intimate or sexual conduct with current service users, students, supervisees, research participants, or with others directly involved in a professional relationship which involves an unequal distribution of power or authority in the social worker's favour (Value 3.4.2e);

- Not to enter into an intimate or sexual relationship with a former service user without careful consideration of any potential for exploitation, taking advice as appropriate (Value 3.4.2f).

More recent government documents also hold some interesting details. Following the death of 'Baby' Peter Connelly in 2007 and subsequent investigations and inquiries, two important reports have been published. The Laming report (Lord Laming 2009) reviewed the government's child protection reforms and made a number of recommendations including that the law should be changed to include senior managers in the registration requirements with the GSCC in order that they also comply with the mandatory code of conduct. The report by Lord Laming, who also chaired the inquiry into the death of Victoria Climbié, did acknowledge the emotional dimension of social work, saying that '[Social workers] need to develop the emotional resilience to manage the challenges they will face in dealing with potentially difficult families'. (Lord Laming 2009:52). However, his report seems to omit other important dimensions, potentially misleading the public and misrepresenting vital information. The report makes no mention of the gender of workers or the majority of their clients (who are mostly women) and his figures seem to greatly underestimate domestic violence. He argues that of the 11 million children in England '200,000 children live in households where there is a known high risk case of domestic abuse and violence' (Lord Laming, 2009:13). As prevalence studies have shown that about 6–10% of women experience domestic violence in any one year (Featherstone 2009, Barter 2009, Mirrlees-Black 1999); 200,000 seems to be a massive underestimate.

Similarly, in another government report published earlier this year, a report which was intended to advise on a comprehensive reform programme for social work, outlining a 'vision' for the profession, there is only one reference to domestic violence and no references to gender, men, women, sex or sexuality (DoH and DfCSF 2009). Neither of the reports refers to other factors relating to gender which may impact on social workers as professionals, for example that one-fifth of British women were sexually abused as children (Goodchild 2007). Both reports also fail to consider personal or relationship factors for staff as relevant to their remit, despite the Task Force report considering the 'calibre of entrants', where they allude to 'emotional resilience' (25) and 'developing skills in … operating in dangerous family environments and dealing with deception, diversion and hostility' (28).

It seems that, on the one hand, the government and our own professional body wish to involve themselves in the regulation and scrutiny of social work conduct; yet, on the other hand, they overlook and avoid fundamental elements of the day-to-day experiences of staff. Neither government guidance on conduct nor codes of ethics and governance have been able to shed much light on how gender and sexuality contribute to social work as a profession, nor do they add any information about what should be regulated regarding personal conduct. Indeed, the codes seem vague, unhelpful and misleading. They make little reference to our relationships with each other and offer no analysis of the significance of gender or sexualities. Who are we and 'how' should we be?

Some illustrations from personal experience

Perhaps my main interest in all of this has arisen because I have spent many years negotiating my own way as a heterosexual feminist in a world where sexuality is, and has always been, a particular site of women's subordination to men (Maynard and Purvis 1995). How I have experienced inequality and discrimination, and how I have understood these experiences, has led me to two inter-related themes about communication and sincerity.

In my experience, communication and power have always played a central role (in my personal and working lives) and these have always seemed to resonate with flirting and humour. A great deal of our communications have a sexual element, often very subtle, and reflecting back on my own experiences as a heterosexual woman, much of my time was spent navigating these exchanges with jokes and innuendos. The ease, or otherwise, of getting through difficult situations, smoothing over angry exchanges, surviving frustrating disappointments and enduring awkward moments, often seemed to relate to the gender and sexuality of the players. Often, what I knew (or felt I knew) about a person, was crucial to the communication and the relationship. No doubt this was reciprocal, what they knew about me would influence their responses to me. But, as Reynolds (2008) asks, 'how do we make personal information about ourselves known to others, and how do we find out about them?' (2008:146).

At a conference about sexuality for social workers a couple of years ago I was asked to lead two workshops about sexual identities and relationships in practice. I asked participants if they would complete a short questionnaire to stimulate thinking and discussion about how we know and find out about each others' sexualities. However, workshop participants were invited to add some personal information if willing (age, gender and sexuality) and leave or return it to me for further analysis. Twenty-six people completed them: 10 heterosexual women and 10 lesbians, 4 gay men and 2 heterosexual men (one described himself as 'predominantly heterosexual' and the other as 'heterosexual so far'). Although most of the workshop participants said they did not ask about their clients' or each others' sexualities, many said that people accurately assumed theirs (especially the heterosexual women). However, most of the lesbians said they had told people themselves, though 2 also said that some people had assumed wrongly. Interestingly, despite their reluctance to ask, almost all the women (9 lesbians and 9 heterosexual women) said they knew or thought they knew their colleagues' sexualities – unlike the men, who did not. Might this difference be replicated amongst other social workers? Are all women better at guessing and/or knowing the sexualities of others than men, or do they just think they are?

Clearly this was not conducted as research and the 'results' cannot be regarded in any reliable way as showing anything other than some interesting ideas. Perhaps one of the most interesting things was that, despite the conference being for experienced social workers and about sexuality, some of the participants were unsure of their own sexual identities. One 50-year-old woman said she didn't know her own sexuality. Should social workers, who are expected to be self-aware and reflective, be unsure or ambiguous about themselves? Might this be true for many of us and is this something more of us should consider, or is it something that seems too difficult to grapple with? If, as the GSCC (2004) requires, practitioners must 'strive to establish and maintain the trust and confidence of service users and carers' (Code 2), should we communicate more confidently in relation to who we are? Surely, in terms of accountability alone, this might be the least we should strive for (Banks 2002).

This leads to the second theme about sincerity. Returning to an influential book mentioned at the beginning of this chapter (Hockey, Meah and Robinson 2007), Hockey and her colleagues found concealment to be a fundamental aspect of heterosexuality (117), discovering many stigmatizing secrets, troubling inconsistencies, anxious silences and distressing instabilities in their participants' heterosexual relationships.

Family members gave contradictory accounts of shared events; generations revealed one another's secrets ... [and] transgressive heterosexuality. Not only was talk of reproductive and sexual matters silenced – evidence of a tension between respectability and sexuality – but also extra-marital relationships (Hockey, Meah and Robinson 2007:116).

As mentioned before, much of my time in social work practice and education has meant I had to think about communication and power, particularly in relation to gender and sexuality with men (almost always heterosexual men) in managerial and regulatory positions. These experiences have sometimes been good and often involved some element of humour and flirting. Some have been less easy and, on reflection, it seems to me that these have been linked to sincerity and honesty. Many times I have known of colleagues' infidelities, use of pornography or violence in their personal relationships, though of course, these behaviours have not been alluded to. These silent aspects of our communications resonate in our relationships and make it difficult, if not impossible for me to employ the usual humour or flirting to help out. Should social workers, who are expected to be honest and trustworthy, engage in such fraudulent exchanges? As the Task Force report considers the 'calibre of entrants' (25), might it also consider these more private and personal aspects of our lives, particularly as it states that social workers are regularly 'dealing with deception' (DoH and DfCSF, 2009:28). How many of us are hiding our personal circumstances and sexual histories, perhaps often wishing we could hide our sexual identities, yet somehow still adhering to social work values? Could it be different?

Talking about personal relationships and sexual matters is something most of us do quite regularly and easily in social gatherings – discussing our friends' relationships, laughing at the sexual exploits of celebrities and sharing our opinions on education policies, health promotions or legal reforms relating to sexuality. We almost certainly all talk about who we know, how we may seem to others and how this affirms (or otherwise) our identity. However, talking about relationships and sexual matters in relation to our work – as a social work practitioner, researcher or educator – seems to be quite a different matter. Despite sexual identity being addressed in terms of anti-discriminatory and diversity agendas, and much of the governance and policy guidance now adhering to diversity policies, most of social work practice, research and education skates over the contradictory dimensions of heterosexuality in the lives of all those involved.

Conclusions

If, in terms of heterosexuality, we only seem to know about the extremes of each others' lives – the mundane and monogamous (which is spoken about) or the deceptive and dangerous (which is silenced) – we cannot relate to each other honestly. If this is true, how are we to accurately assess and justly direct others' lives? In parallel to these anomalies in our experiences, what are the omissions and inaccuracies in the literature and government documents about personal and professional dimensions of social work practice in relation to heterosexuality? These discrepancies must be addressed. Social work research and education need to revisit feminist understandings of heterosexuality and incorporate these more centrally in their endeavours. Documents relating to conduct and governance should be re-written in order that they might more honestly account for the realities of heterosexual life, and heterosexual social workers (both women and men) might offer some solutions by being more truthful about personal issues in their professional practice. A great deal could be achieved by drawing on feminist literature and understandings to help us decipher the broader meanings of sexuality. This in turn might enable us to re-orient the sexual self with the personal, every-day realm of experience and address it in a more comprehensive and sincere way.

References

Adams, R., Dominelli, L. & Payne, M. (Editors) 2002. *Critical Practice in Social Work*. Basingstoke: Palgrave.

Ault, A. & Brzuzy, S. 2009. Removing gender identity disorder from the Diagnostic and Statistical Manual of Mental Disorders: a call for action. *Social Work*, 54(2), 187–189.

Balen, R. & Crawshaw, M. (Editors) 2006. *Sexuality and Fertility Issues in Ill Health and Disability*. London: Jessica Kingsley.

Banks, S. 2002. 'Professional values and accountabilities', in *Critical Practice in Social Work*, edited by R. Adams, L. Dominelli & M. Payne. Basingstoke: Palgrave, 28–37.

Barlow, C. and Hall, B.L. 2007. 'What about feelings?' A study of emotion and tension in social work field education. *Social Work Education*, 26(4), 399–413.

Barter, C. 2009. In the name of love: partner abuse and violence in teenage relationships. *British Journal of Social Work*, 39(2), 211–233.

BASW 2006. *Code of Ethics for Social Work* [online]. http://basw.co.uk [accessed 14.9.06].

Biestek, F.P. 1989. *The Casework Relationship.* 12th Edition. London: Unwin Hyman Ltd.

Bornat, J., Johnson, J., Pereira, C., Pilgrim, D. & Williams, F. (Editors) 1997. *Community Care: A Reader*. Basingstoke: Macmillan.

Brand, J. 2009. The death of good practice? *Professional Social Work*, October 2009, 10–11.

Bremner, J. & Hillin, A. 1994. *Sexuality, Young People and Care: Creating Positive Contexts for Training, Policy and Development*. Lyme Regis: Russell House Publishing.

Burman, E. 2009. Beyond 'emotional literacy' in feminist and educational research. *British Educational Research Journal*, 35(1), 137–155.

Butler, G. 2007. Reflecting on emotion in social work, in *Reflective Practice in Social Work*, edited by C. Knott and T. Scragg. Exeter: Learning Matters, 33–47.

Cant, B. 2006. Exploring the implications for health professionals of men coming out as gay in healthcare settings. *Health and Social Care in the Community*, 14(1), 9–16.

Carabine, J. 2004. Personal lives, public policies and normal sexualities?, in *Sexualities: Personal Lives and Social Policy*, edited by J. Carabine. Bristol: Policy Press, 1–48.

Carter, P. and Jeffs, T. 1995. *A Very Private Affair: Sexual Exploitation in Higher Education*. Derbyshire: Education Now Books.

Charles, H. 1993. 'A homogeneous habit? Heterosexual display in the English holiday camp', in *Heterosexuality: A Feminism and Psychology Reader*, edited by S. Wilkinson & C. Kitzinger. London: Sage, 270–272.

Christie, A. 2001. (Editor) *Men and Social Work: Theories and Practices*. Basingstoke: Palgrave.

Christie, A. 2006. Negotiating the uncomfortable intersections between gender and professional identities in social work. *Critical Social Policy*, 26(2), 390–411.

Cincotta, N., Childs, J. & Eichenfield, A. 2006. Sexuality and growing up HIV-positive: lessons from practice, in *Sexuality and Fertility Issues in Ill Health and Disability*, edited by R. Balen & M. Crawshaw. London: Jessica Kingsley, 206–220.

Coffey, A. 2002 Sex in the field: intimacy and intimidation, in *Ethical Dilemmas in Qualitative Research*, edited by T. Welland & L. Pugsley. Aldershot: Ashgate, 57–74.

Collander-Brown, D. 2005. Being with another as a professional practitioner: uncovering the nature of working with individuals. *Youth and Policy*, 86, Winter, 33–47.

Cooper, A. & Lousada, J. 2005. *Borderline Welfare: Feeling and Fear of Feeling in Modern Welfare.* London: Karnac.

Cosis Brown, H. 1998. *Social Work and Sexuality: Working with Lesbians and Gay Men.* Basingstoke: Macmillan.

Cox, P., Kershaw, S. & Trotter, J. 2000. *Child Sexual Assault: Feminist Perspectives.* Basingstoke: Palgrave.

Cull, M. 2006. Dispelling the taboo of intersex conditions: we're only human like you, in *Sexuality and Fertility Issues in Ill Health and Disability*, edited by R. Balen and M. Crawshaw. London: Jessica Kingsley, 192–205.

Dickson-Swift, V., James, E.L., Kippen, S. & Liamputtong, P. 2009. Researching sensitive topics: qualitative research as emotion work. *Qualitative Research*, 9(1), 61–79.

DoH and DfCSF 2009. *Facing Up To The Task: The interim report of the Social Work Task Force.* [Online]. http://publications.dcsf.gov.uk [accessed 31.7.09].

Dominelli, L. 2002. Glassed-in: Problematising women's reproductive rights under the new reproductive technologies, in *Critical Practice in Social Work*, edited by R. Adams, L. Dominelli & M. Payne. Basingstoke: Palgrave, 72–80.

Dunk, P. 2007. Everyday sexuality and social work: locating sexuality in professional practice and education. *Social Work and Society*, 5(2), 135–142.

Featherstone, B. 2009. *Contemporary Fathering: Theory, Policy and Practice.* Bristol: Policy Press.

Fenge, L-A. & Fannin, A. 2009. Sexuality and bereavement: implications for practice with older lesbians and gay men. *Practice: Social Work in Action*, 21(1), 35–46.

Ferguson, H. 2005 Working with violence, the emotions and the psycho-social dynamics of child protection: reflections on the Victoria Climbie Case. *Social Work Education*, 24(7), 781–795.

Fish, J. 2009. Invisible no more? Including lesbian, gay and bisexual people in social work and social care. *Practice: Social Work in Action*, 21(1), 47–64.

Fraser, H. 2005. Women, love, and intimacy 'gone wrong': fire, wind, and ice. *Affilia*, 29(1), 10–20.

Freel, M. 2003. Child sexual abuse and the male monopoly: an empirical exploration of gender and a sexual interest in children. *British Journal of Social Work*, 33(4), 481–498.

Frith, H. & Gleeson, K. 2004. Clothing and embodiment: men managing body image and appearance. *Psychology of Men and Masculinity*, 5(1), 40–4.

Goodchild, S. 2007 One fifth of British women were sexually abused as children. *The Independent on Sunday*, 1 April, 2.

Green, L., Butt, T. & King, N. 2002. Taking the chaste out of chastisement: an analysis of the sexual implications of the corporal punishment of children. *Childhood*, 9(2), 205–224.

GSCC 2004. *Code of Practice for Social Care Workers and Code of Practice for Employers of Social Care Workers*. London: The Stationary Office.

GSCC 2009a. Newsletter: Messages from conduct hearings [Online: Social Work Connections]. http://www.socialworkconnections.org.uk/ [accessed 28.7.09].

GSCC 2009b. Social workers: analysis of GSCC registration and qualifications data, *Analysis Notes*, Volume 2d: North East. June 2009.

Guy, A., Green, E. & Banim, M. 2001. (Editors) *Through the Wardrobe: Women's Relationships with their Clothes*. Oxford: Berg.

Harding, R. & Hamilton, P. 2009. Working girls: abuse or choice in street-level sex work? A study of homeless women in Nottingham. *British Journal of Social Work*, 39(6), 1118–1137.

Hargreaves, D. A. & Tiggemann, M. 2006. 'Body image is for girls': a qualitative study of boys' body image. *Journal of Health Psychology*, 11(4), 567–576.

Hayes, P. & Campbell, J. 2005. *Bloody Sunday: Trauma, Pain and Politics*. London: Pluto Press.

Hearn, J. & Pringle, K. 2006. Men, masculinities and children: some European perspectives. *Critical Social Policy*, 26(2), 365–389.

Hicks, S. 2001. Men social workers in children's services: 'will the *real man* please stand up?', in *Men and Social Work: Theories and Practices*, edited by A. Christie. Basingstoke: Palgrave. Pages 49–62.

Hicks, S. 2008. What does social work desire? *Social Work Education*, 27(2), 131–137.

Hirst, G. & Cox, P. 1996. Hearing all sides of the story: the challenge of integrating teaching on sexual aggression into social work qualifying training. *The Journal of Sexual Aggression*, 2(1), 33–48.

Hockey, J., Meah, A. & Robinson, V. 2007. *Mundane Heterosexualities: From Theory to Practices*. Basingstoke: Palgrave Macmillan.

Hugman, R. (2009) But is it social work? Some reflections on mistaken identities. *British Journal of Social Work*, 39, 1138–1153.

Karban, K. (2007) Book Review: Sexual Issues in Social Work. *British Journal of Social Work*, 37(8), 1442–1444.

Keery H., Boutelle, K., van den Berg, P. & Thompson, J.K. 2005. The impact of appearance-related teasing by family members. *Journal of Adolescent Health*, 37(2), 120–127.

Kirkman, M., Rosenthal, D.A. and Fieldman, S.S. 2005. Being open with your mouth shut: the meaning of 'openness' in family communication about sexuality. *Sex Education: Sexuality, Society and Learning*, 5(1), 49–66.

Kitzinger, C. 2005. Heteronormativity in action: reproducing the heterosexual nuclear family in 'after hours' medical calls. *Social Problems*, 52 (4), 477–498.

Knott, C. & Scragg, T. 2007. (Editors) *Reflective Practice in Social Work*. Exeter: Learning Matters.

Leech, N. & Trotter, J. 2005. 'None of them ever asked about sex': some personal thoughts as to why social workers have difficulty discussing sexuality with young people. *Socio-analysis*, 7, 19–36.

Leech, N. & Trotter, J. 2006. Alone and together: some thoughts on reflective learning for work with adult survivors of child sexual abuse. *The Journal of Social Work Practice*, 20(2), 175–187.

Logan, J. & Kershaw, S. 1994 Heterosexism and social work education: the invisible challenge. *Social Work Education*, 13(3), 61–80.

Lord Laming 2009. *The Protection of Children in England: A Progress Report.* London: The Stationary Office.

Lovelock, R., Lyons, K. & Powell, J. 2004. (Editors) *Reflecting on Social Work: Discipline and Profession*. Aldershot: Ashgate.

Lyons, K. & Taylor, I. 2004 Gender and knowledge in social work in *Reflecting on Social Work: Discipline and Profession*, edited by R. Lovelock, K. Lyons & J. Aldershot: Ashgate, 72–94.

Mackinnon, J. 2004. Academic supervision: seeking metaphors and models for equality. *Journal of Further and Higher Education*, 28(4), 395–405.

Marlowe, C.M., Schneider, S.L. & Nelson, C.E. 1996. Gender and attractiveness biases in hiring decisions: Are more experienced managers less biased? *Journal of Applied Psychology*, 81, 11–21.

Maynard, M. and Purvis, J. 1995. (Editors) *(Hetero)sexual Politics*. London: Taylor and Francis.

Milward, R. 2008. *Apples*. London: Faber and Faber.

Mirrlees-Black, C. 1999. *Domestic Violence: Findings from a New British Crime Survey Self-completion Questionnaire*. London: Home Office.

Moon, J.A. 2004. *A Handbook of Reflective and Experiential Learning: Theory and Practice*. London: RoutledgeFalmer.

Morris, J. 1997. 'Us' and 'them'? Feminist research and community care, in *Community Care: A Reader*, edited by J. Bornat, J. Johnson, C. Pereira, D. Pilgrim & F. Williams. Basingstoke: Macmillan, 160–167.

Morrison, T. 2007. Emotional intelligence, emotion and social work: context, characteristics, complications and contribution. *British Journal of Social Work*, 37, 245–263.

Mullender, A. 2002. Persistent oppressions: the example of domestic violence, in *Critical Practice in Social Work*, edited by R. Adams, L. Dominelli & M. Payne. Basingstoke: Palgrave, 63–71.

Myers, S. 2008. Revisiting Lancaster: more things that every social work student should know. *Social Work Education*, 27(2), 203–211.

National Lesbian and Gay Survey 1992. *What a Lesbian Looks Like: Writings by Lesbians on their Lives and Lifestyles*. London: Routledge.

O'Connell Davidson, J. 1995. British sex tourists in Thailand, in *(Hetero)sexual Politics*, edited by M. Maynard & J. Purvis. London: Taylor and Francis, 42–64.

Orme, J. 2001. *Gender and Community Care: Social Work and Social Care Perspectives*. Basingstoke: Palgrave.

Paechter, C. 2007. *Being Boys, Being Girls: Learning Masculinities and Femininities*. Maidenhead: Open University Press.

Plummer, K. 2001. *Documents of Life: An Invitation to Critical Humanism.* London: Sage.

Pugh, R. 2007. Dual relationships: personal and professional boundaries in rural social work. *British Journal of Social Work*, 37, 1405–1423.

Raudenbush, B. & Zellner, D.A. 1997. Nobody's satisfied: effects of abnormal eating behaviors and actual and perceived weight status on body image satisfaction in males and females. *Journal of Social and Clinical Psychology*, 16, 95–110.

Reynolds, J. 2008. *The Single Woman: A Discursive Investigation.* Hove: Routledge.

Ruch, G. 2005. Relationship-based and reflective practice: holistic approaches to contemporary child care social work. *Child and Family Social Work*, 10, 111–123.

Ryan, A.B. 2001. *Feminist Ways of Knowing: Towards Theorising the Person for Radical Adult Education.* Leicester: NIACE.

Satterly, B. 2004. The intention and reflection model: gay male therapist self-disclosure and identity management. *Journal of Lesbian and Gay Social Services*, 17(4), 69–86.

Scourfield, J. 2003. *Gender and Child Protection.* Basingstoke: Palgrave.

Shaw, A. 2008. Book review, *Professional Social Work*, Birmingham: BASW.

Shernoff, M. 2004. Barebacking and challenges to therapeutic neutrality. *Journal of Lesbian and Gay Social Services*, 17(4), 59–68.

Shildrick, M. 2004. Silencing sexuality: the regulation of the disabled body, in *Sexualities: Personal Lives and Social Policy*, edited by J. Carabine. Bristol: Policy Press, 123–157.

Smart, C. 2007. *Personal Life.* Cambridge: Polity Press.

Smethurst, C. 2007. Gender and reflective practice, in *Reflective Practice in Social Work*, edited by C. Knott and T. Scragg. Exeter: Learning Matters, 91–101.

Stevens, M., Manthorpe, J., Martineau, S., Hussein, S., Rapaport, J. & Harris, J. 2008. Making decisions about who should be barred from working with adults in vulnerable situations: the need for social work understanding. *British Journal of Social Work*, Advance Access, October 1st 2010, doi:10.1093/bjsw/bcn135.

Swanberg, J.E. and Macke, C. 2006. Intimate partner violence and the workplace: consequences and disclosure. *Affilia*, 21(4), 391–406.

Trotter, J. 2001. Challenging assumptions around sexuality: services for young people. *Youth and Policy*, 71, 25–43.

Trotter, J. 2006a. *Communicating Honestly: Personal Identity and Professional Practice.* Paper to the Sexuality in Social Work and Social Care Conference, London, 20 October 2006.

Trotter, J. 2006b. Violent crimes? Young people's experiences of homophobia and misogyny in secondary schools. *Practice: Social Work in Action*, 18(4), 291–302.

Trotter, J., Crawley, M., Duggan, L., Foster, E. & Levie, J. 2009. Reflecting on what? 'PQ', portfolios and personal issues. *Practice: Social Work in Action*, 21(1), 5–15.

Trotter, J., Kershaw, S. & Knott, C. 2008. Editorial: updating all our outfits. *Social Work Education*, 27(2), 1–5.

Wallis, S. 2007. Reflection and avoiding professional dangerousness in *Reflective Practice in Social Work*, edited by C. Knott & T. Scragg. Exeter: Learning Matters, 79–90.

Welland, T. & Pugsley, L. 2002. (Editors) *Ethical Dilemmas in Qualitative Research*. Aldershot: Ashgate.

White, V. 2006. *The State of Feminist Social Work*. London: Routledge.

Winn, J. & Nutt, D. 2001. From closet to wardrobe?, in *Through the Wardrobe: Women's Relationships with their Clothes*, edited by A. Guy, E. Green & M. Banim. Oxford: Berg, 221–236.

Yacoub, E. & Hall, I. 2007. The sexual lives of men with mild learning disability: a qualitative study. *British Journal of Learning Disabilities*, 37(1), 5–11.

Zaidel, D.W., Aarde, S.M. & Baig, K. 2005. Appearance of symmetry, beauty, and health in human faces. *Brain and Cognition*, 57, 261–263.

Chapter 9
Sexuality before Ability?
The Assessment of Lesbians as Adopters

Christine Cocker

[...] well I shall tell them, I shall tell them you're my mums, and I love you, and you're the best thing that could have happened to me.

Isobel, quoting her adopted son, John (age 11).

Introduction

There is increasing interest from adoption agencies in assessing lesbians and gay men. However whilst there have been a number of articles written about lesbian and gay adoption and fostering over recent years (Brown 1991, Hicks 1996, Hicks 1997, Hicks and McDermott 1999, Hicks 2000, Logan and Sellick 2007, Hicks 2005a, Hicks 2005b, Hicks 2008, Brown and Cocker 2008, Cocker and Brown 2010), there is an absence of UK based empirical research about the particular issues and challenges adoption assessments raise from the perspective of lesbians and gay men themselves. Indeed, there is little research available about the efficacy of the adoption assessment process generally, and no existing research that examines the numbers of lesbian and gay prospective adoption applicants, the outcomes of their assessments, and of any adoption placements made with them, although there is now some national data available on numbers of lesbian and gay adopters who have successfully adopted children (DCSF 2007, DCSF 2008, DCSF 2009, Stott 2009).

This chapter discusses the results of a small qualitative study[1] undertaken during 2009, where eleven lesbians who had successfully adopted children were interviewed about their experiences of adoption assessments. This builds on earlier studies where qualitative methods were used to investigate the experiences of lesbian and gay adopters (Skeates and Jabri 1988, Hicks 1996, 1997, 1998, Hicks and McDermott 1999). The aims for this project were threefold: firstly, to explore lesbian adopters' experiences of their assessments; secondly, to consider how the adoption assessment experience prepared adopters to make decisions about adoption; and thirdly, to examine how issues specific to the homosexuality

1   I would like to thank all the women who gave up their time to be interviewed for this study. This study was funded through the CETL linked to the Department of Mental Health and Social Work at Middlesex University, London.

of the adopters were raised and discussed within the assessment process. This is relevant because the social, political and legal framework has changed markedly over the past ten years in relation to the protection that lesbians and gay men now have under the law. This has been commented on elsewhere (Fish 2007, Brown and Kershaw 2008, Bagilhole 2009, Cocker and Hafford Letchfield 2010).

In the UK the Adoption and Children Act 2002 and the Equality Act (Sexual Orientation) Regulations 2007 are fundamentally important in two ways. Firstly, the 2007 Regulations ensure that lesbians and gay men have the same access to assessment at any local authority or independent adoption agency as any other applicant. This is not to say that any applicant, regardless of sexuality, has an automatic right or entitlement to adopt; rather, prospective applicants have the right to request an assessment. However, suitability is determined on the basis of the needs of any child requiring placement, and decision-making occurs with the child's needs taking priority above all else. Secondly, the 2002 legislation offers lesbian and gay couples the opportunity to jointly adopt children. Cocker and Brown (2010) suggest that this has had an effect on Adoption Agencies, who needed to re-think their recruitment strategies. Word-of-mouth is already known to be a powerful aid to recruitment of adopters and foster carers (Fostering Network 2006); therefore if lesbian and gay men have positive experiences of agencies' assessments, this will have a snowballing effect, and those agencies will be approached by other lesbians and gay men interested in adoption.

Literature review

There are a number of books (Brown 1998, Hicks and McDermott 1999, Brown and Cocker 2011), articles (Hicks 2005a, Logan and Sellick 2007, Hicks 2008, Brown and Cocker 2008, Cocker and Brown 2010) and practice guidance or specialist texts (Mallon and Betts 2005, Hicks et al. 2007, Hill 2009) that provide a comprehensive overview of developments in fostering and adoption with lesbians and gay men. Some limited primary research has been undertaken with lesbian and gay prospective adopters and foster carers in the UK, and this is summarized below.

There are a range of systematic reviews and longitudinal research projects that examine outcomes for children growing up in lesbian households (Golombok et al. 1983, Tasker and Golombok 1991 and 1997, Tasker 1999, Patterson 2005). Studies involving children growing up with gay fathers are less common (Patterson 2004, Barrett and Tasker 2001 and 2002, Tasker 2005). In the UK, Golombok's longitudinal studies have been fundamentally important in providing evidence about the differences and similarities between children growing up in lesbian families compared with children growing up in heterosexual single parent (female) families. One of the limitations of these studies is that they are reductionist in nature – they look for problems and negative differences between children of lesbian parents and single female heterosexual parents by asking whether the outcomes for these children are 'as good as' those raised within heterosexual families . Nevertheless, Golombok's study shows that outcomes for the children raised within lesbian households are just as good as the outcomes for children with a heterosexual mother. The sexual orientation of the parent makes little (if any) difference to the outcomes for children. Golombok argues, 'it is what happens within families, not the way families are composed, that seems to matter most' (Golombok 2000:101). As important as this research is, another of its flaws is that it was not designed to enable a more complex understanding of the ways in which non-heterosexual family structures work. It did not specifically review or address the ways in which lesbians become parents (i.e. through heterosexual relationships; donor insemination with a known father; donor insemination using a clinic; or via fostering; kinship arrangements; adoption; or other route). These gaps remain.

Fostering and adoption: primary research with lesbians and gay men

There is very little primary research available which looks at outcomes for children in public care placed with lesbian and gay adopters. There are still relatively small numbers of lesbians and gay men who adopt children. It is only in the last three years that the DCSF has begun collecting annual data about the number of adoptions involving lesbian and gay adopters (see Table 1).

The National Adoption Register, co-ordinated by the British Association of Adoption and Fostering (BAAF) contains some information about the numbers of lesbian or gay approved adopters who have been added to the register and matched with a child/children, and the length of time they have had to wait (Stott 2009).

There is a little more known about the experiences of lesbian or gay prospective and adopters in the UK. Hicks (2005a) provides a summary of some of the earlier research undertaken over the past 20 years, also comprising small-scale qualitative interviews. Skeates and Jabri (1988) was the first UK publication to address lesbian and gay fostering and adoption practices. Their research highlighted the existence of discriminatory ideas about lesbians and gay men within social welfare organizations, and showed the problems lesbians and gay men experienced when being assessed as prospective adopters. Of the thirteen people involved in this study, ten were 'out' to their assessing social worker, three were not; those that were open about their sexuality reported difficulties in the way in which the agency viewed their sexuality. For those who successfully completed the assessment, a disproportionate number were then matched with disabled children, which Parmar refers to as sending out messages of 'second class children for second class carers' (Parmar 1989, cited in Hicks 2005a:44).

Hicks also conducted small-scale qualitative research investigating lesbian and gay prospective adopters' experience of the adoption assessment (Hicks 1993, 1996, 1997 and 1998) as well as examining the experience of social workers undertaking such assessments (Hicks 2000). Hicks' earlier studies (1993 and 1996) raised similar issues to those uncovered by Skeates and Jabri (1988), including: whether or not prospective adopters or foster carers should be out as

Table 9.1   Children looked after who were adopted during the years ending 31 March by number of adopters, legal status of adopters and by gender of adopters[1] (years ending 31 March 2007 to 2009; coverage: England).

	Numbers			Percentages		
	2007	2008	2009	2007	2008	2009
All children looked after who were adopted during the year ending 31 March	3,300	3,200	3,300	100	100	100
Number of adopters	3,300	3,200	3,300	100	100	100
1 person	290	270	270	9	9	8
2 persons	3,000	2,900	3,000	91	91	92
Legal status and gender of adopters	3,300	3,200	3,300	100	100	100
Single adopter	290	270	270	9	9	8
Single male adopter	20	10	10	1	0	0
Single female adopter	280	260	260	8	8	8
Same sex couple not in civil partnership	70	50	50	2	2	1
Adopting couple are both male	20	20	20	0	1	1
Adopting couple are both female	60	30	30	2	1	1
Different sex unmarried couple	150	140	190	4	5	6
Civil partnership couple	20	30	80	1	1	2
Adopting couple are both male	10	–	40	0	–	1
Adopting couple are both female	10	20	40	0	1	1
Married couple	2,800	2,700	2,700	84	84	82

Source: SSDA 903

1   Historical data may differ from older publications. This is mainly due to the implementation of amendments and corrections sent by some local authorities after the publication date of previous materials.

openly gay or lesbian for fear of being rejected; a fear of media intrusion (Hicks and McDermott 1999); once approved, lesbian and gay foster carers reported waiting longer for placements; the vast majority of these placements were either short-term or emergency placements, or they were not used at all; and, when they were used, the majority of foster carers had disabled children placed with them (Hicks 2005a:45). Hicks (1998) also reported that adoption by lesbians and gay men was rare at the time, because of agencies' reluctance to place young children in lesbian or gay households, and because adoption panels did not approve the match.

The main themes reported by prospective adopters in studies Hicks undertook in 1996 and 1997 included: social work agencies rejecting prospective adopters outright or 'making discriminatory statements about sexuality; assessing social workers having limited knowledge about lesbian or gay lives or, in some cases, avoiding discussion of their sexuality altogether; concerns about the gender role models that lesbians or gay men would provide; and, a fear that gay men, in particular, might sexually abuse children' (Hicks 2005a:47–48). Hicks' work showed that lesbian and gay applications were subject to tougher forms of scrutiny than others. Hicks and McDermott (1999) recount the experiences of seventeen adopters and foster carers in the UK who had looked after children placed with them. Again, what emerged from this study were the additional hurdles that lesbian and gay foster carers and adopters faced and were expected to negotiate, from the assessing agency, any community agencies involved with the child (such as schools) and workplace negotiations, e.g. regarding adoption leave.

There is more literature available from USA concerning the experiences of lesbian and gay prospective adopters and foster carers, as well as the outcomes for children adopted and fostered by lesbians and gay men. This shows that lesbian adopters are broadly satisfied with their overall adoption experience (Ryan and Whitlock 2009), an adoptive parent's sexual orientation is not a significant factor in terms of the outcomes for the child or children placed with families (Erich et al. 2009), that lesbian and gay adoptive families have good levels of support from their networks (Erich 2005, Kindle et al. 2005), and that outcomes are especially good for older children placed with lesbian or gay adopters (Erich 2005, Leung et al. 2005).

In terms of the ability of lesbian and gay adopters to successfully parent children, these results broadly concur with the findings of Golombok's work with lesbians parenting birth children. However, there may be differences in the kinds of children that lesbian or gay adopters are looking to adopt. Stott (2009) indicated that there may be differences between lesbian and gay adopters and other adopters regarding the type of children they would consider for adoption (Cocker and Anderson 2011). Of course another explanation for these differences may well be that lesbians and gay men keep their options as open as possible in terms of the kind of child that they would like to parent, because of potential difficulties (and these may be real or perceived by the adopters themselves) for lesbian or gay adopters being matched to children. In other words, do they still wait longer than heterosexual carers? Are lesbian or gay adopters or foster carers more likely to be matched with disabled children as they were 20 years ago? This requires further investigation.

Fostering and adoption: primary research involving assessing social workers

Hicks has undertaken two separate studies which have involved a number of interviews with assessing social workers (1998, 2000). In the second study (Hicks 2000) suggested that the assessing social workers understood lesbianism through a heteronormative lens, and in-so-doing created three 'types' of 'good' and 'bad' lesbians, with associated virtues, (the 'man-hater', the 'militant' and the 'pedestal of virtue'), and this categorization had a major impact on the assessed applicant's suitability. The lesbians that were most likely to be approved as foster carers or adopters, were:

> able to deal with anti-lesbian prejudices of birth families, some children / young people and panel; were not threatening to gender norms; were integrated with heterosexuals; … likely to know men, have male role models, present positive images of men; be integrated into the wider (heterosexual) community and family; … where child care abilities were emphasized as paramount, over issues of sexuality; were non-militant, non-radical, not political, not too 'feminist....' (Hicks 2000:164),

Logan and Sellick suggest that the debate has now moved:

> [...] from whether or not lesbians and gay men are suitable as carers, to a more critical examination of the process of their becoming approved, and the extent to which social work practice continues to reinforce and perpetuate the superiority of heterosexuality (Logan and Sellick 2007:42).

They suggest, as do others (Dugmore and Cocker 2008, Brown and Cocker 2008, and Cocker and Hafford Letchfield 2010) that the legal changes may not be enough to change social attitudes, including the attitudes and opinions of social workers. But they go on to comment that, 'within a wider context of prejudice and stereotypes, social workers may be left not knowing how to work with lesbian and gay applicants' (2007:42). However, whilst there are a number of practice guidance now available (see below), Brown comments that:

> In my experience capable social work practitioners work capably with all service users and carers and, similarly, incompetent ones work incompetently with all. This is not to say that we should therefore ignore issues of sexuality but rather to argue that social work needs to 'up its game' with some degree of urgency to better the quality of social work practice generally. This relates to two particular areas: social work practitioners' ability to understand and use effectively social work knowledge and, second, that they have the skills to engage with service users and carers effectively in such a way that they are able to effect change (Brown 2008:270).

But how do you change attitudes and practice of staff in this area? Dugmore and Cocker (2008) ran a series of one-day workshops for fostering and adoption social workers on lesbian and gay issues relevant for their work, following the many legislative changes mentioned above. The result of the tests and evaluations that were run pre and post-training (including Hudson and Ricketts (1980) 'Index of Attitudes towards Homosexuals') suggested that workers welcomed the opportunity to discuss these issues within their work, but the delivery of one day's training did not significantly change attitudes.

Practice guidance and practice models

The general assessment process for adoption applicants in England has been documented elsewhere (DH 2003, DFES 2006, Lord 2008, Cocker and Anderson 2011). There are currently two practice guidance documents in circulation (Mallon and Betts 2005, Hicks et al. 2007) that have been written to support the work of the assessing social worker when undertaking home study reports with lesbians and gay applicants. There is, however, some debate about whether the production of such practice guides and frameworks detailing best practice when working with lesbians and gay men and their families, or specialist books for lesbian or gay prospective adoption applicants (Hill 2009) are useful (see Hicks 2008), or whether they are in themselves reductionist because of the normative position they unconsciously or consciously adopt. Cocker and Hafford-Letchfield comment (2010):

> There are occasions when certain types of assessments do need to cover different areas, because some experiences are particular to the lives of lesbians and gay men, for example of coming out or homophobia. The question is whether existing frameworks should be flexible enough to adapt to people's individuality, and incorporate differences in a reflexive manner rather than as an 'add on' or not address them at all.

Cocker and Brown (2010), building on the work of Brown (1991) and Brown and Cocker (2008), have developed a practice model that enables the consideration of sex and sexuality within the assessment process. This model is relevant to all prospective adopters, not just lesbians and gay men. There are concerns rightly expressed about the 'normalization' of the adoption assessment process for all (Logan and Sellick 2007) and the 'equality equals sameness' approach that has featured within social work practice during the last decade or so. Instead, a move toward acknowledging the differences that exist between different people's experiences, whether that is about being lesbian or gay, and/or black, and/or having a disability, is more appropriate. This is not to set in motion a recreation of the 'hierarchy of oppressions' model located in the anti-discriminatory practice discourse (Brown and Cocker 2011), but to acknowledge the skills required when working with difference and complexity, which all social workers should be using capably in their practice.

Methods

For this exploratory study, ethical approval was obtained via Middlesex University. I used semi-structured interviews as the method for collecting data. The questions I asked in each interview corresponded with the initial three aims of the project, which were stated at the beginning of the chapter. Although I had listed a number of questions under each of the three areas of the study, I did not follow the schedule in a strict order. Once the interview had begun, specific questions were asked if the participants didn't cover the subject area of that question during the interview. This ensured that the interview flowed, and the stories of the participants were coherently told. At the beginning of the interview I asked a number of background questions specifically about the living circumstances of the families: for example, who lived in the house; did people work; whether people had had a civil partnership. The interviews were also recorded and transcribed. For the purposes of this chapter, thematic analysis was used to collate, highlight and code topics and sub-topics emerging from the interviews. The results of this are presented below.

The sample

The sample used was a convenience sample, recruited from a number of sources, including an advertisement on the website of a national voluntary organization for lesbian and gay foster carers and adopters; and a number of local authorities who had previously successfully assessed lesbian adopters.

I interviewed eleven women, representing seven families: three families lived in London and four families lived in various small towns in England. All the adopters were in relationships, ranging from ten years to 35 years in duration. All lived with their children, with no other adults or extended family or friends living in the home.

Five families had adopted under the old adoption legislation (Adoption Act 1976), and two adopted under the new legislation (Adoption and Children Act 2002). One woman had been assessed under both Acts in order that she could have the same legal relationship with her adopted child as her partner, rather than having parental responsibility via a joint residence order (Section 8, Children Act 1989) that would end when the child turned 18. One couple had been successfully approved as foster carers, and had fostered their child before adopting him, and this required an adoption assessment from a different agency. The adoptions occurred from 1998 through to 2007.

A total of seven children (four girls and three boys) had been adopted by the families taking part in the study. All but one of the children were under four years of age at the time the placement began, with the majority of children aged under two at the time of placement. Five children are white British, one child is white and black British, and one child is Asian. Two children have learning disabilities, and the majority of other children had experienced difficulties in school, with some receiving additional support via Special Educational Needs (SEN) services. Three families have also received specialist Child and Adolescent Mental Health Services (CAMHS) support because of the particular needs of their child.

I interviewed four couples together and three women without their partner being present. One of the couples and two of the women I interviewed had other birth children, who were all older than their adopted child, and one woman had parented a child in a previous relationship who was not her birth child, and this child was now an adult. Five couples had a civil partnership or equivalent. All of the women I interviewed were white (four were white European), and ranged in age from mid-thirties to mid-fifties. The partner of one woman I interviewed was British Asian. All, except two women, regularly worked in paid employment. The two other women worked occasionally. The names used in this study are pseudonyms chosen by the participants.

Results

This was a retrospective study so I relied on people's memory of the assessment, including dates. Two women had kept diaries so were able to provide dates, times and places for everything I asked about. However, even without these specifics, the level of detail that participants remembered about the process they had gone through was considerable.

The adopters' experiences of their assessing agency:

In terms of the assessment process overall, all except one couple recounted a broadly positive experience of the agency they had chosen to conduct their assessment. Additionally the participant who had been through two assessments was able to compare the two authorities, and she was more critical of the second authority's assessment, which had occurred under the new legislation. All recounted a similar process of assessment, comprising: a home study report; a preparation group with other prospective adopters; presentation at panel, with the majority of participants attending panel; the matching process with a further panel attendance; introductions; and placement.

In terms of participants' initial contact with agencies, it was clear that all except one couple had done their 'homework' in terms of gathering information and making enquiries. The couple who hadn't had a choice about the agency they approached had fostered their child prior to adopting him: this agency assessed them. Most people used a combination of 'word of mouth' – approaching agencies that either had good reputations for working with lesbians and gay men, or had advertised in the lesbian and gay press, or rang a number of agencies and then approached the agency where they got the best response. The majority of participants said that their initial contact with their chosen agency was positive, although a few people recounted being given a grilling by the social workers they met, about their motivation to adopt.

> *Cecelia* – We chose that agency because they had a fairly positive reputation for assessing lesbians and gay men and we didn't want to be guinea pigs for a local authority that was new to assessing lesbians and gay men. We approached 3 Local Authorities. One never got back to us despite contacting (them) a few times even though they are supposed to be an excellent social services department. Another one we did make contact with after seeing them advertise in the gay press, and a social worker came round but seemed to give us a message that there would be a restriction on the type of child we would be matched with i.e. an older child and that didn't feel very comfortable. One of the reasons for choosing the local authority we did was that the adoption team responded immediately to a phone call with some information about their team and made an appointment fairly promptly for us to go down and have our first visit with them.

> *Jenny* – So I rang them and got, overall quite a positive response. In that first phone call, I did very explicitly ask, 'Have you assessed same sex couples before?' and, I asked her explicitly about what to expect and whether, you know, we would be treated the same way or whether there would be more complications for us … And she said, 'Well we would assess you as fairly as we could as anyone else, but you should probably expect some resistance along the way, could be at matching phase, there could be panel members, could be the other social workers that you have to engage with, that's where you might come across …' erm, I guess she didn't say 'homophobia', but something along the lines of, 'well, people might not exactly understand your kind of family, or that you will have to do some more explaining'.

In terms of the preparation group, participants' experiences were also generally positive. Sessions were sensitively run, with thought given to the needs of the lesbian and gay participants. The majority of participants were not the only lesbian or gay applicants in their preparation group. Some participants talked about the different reasons for people wanting to adopt significantly affecting dynamics in these sessions:

> *Jenny* – Actually throughout the whole preparation group – people's fertility issues – it was just a nightmare because it just kept coming up … not the two single women because they also hadn't wanted to try to get pregnant, they chose adoption instead as their first choice of having a child … all the other couples had much more of an issue with that (fertility) and it kept coming up and it was just a bit detracting from … yeah, it was a bit like a therapy for people who wanted

their birth children, and I think it might have been better if they had done the 'getting over you not having birth children issues' session before the preparation group so people were more ready to actually really focus on adoption ... I think that might have been a better idea.

Regarding the participants' relationship with the assessing social worker, there was overwhelming agreement that this is what made the difference in terms of people's experience of the assessment. All except two people were very positive about their assessing social worker, and there was agreement across the participants interviewed in this study about the skills that really mattered in their relationship with the assessing social worker:

Lily – With experience they know what they are doing. Um and I think there's a sort of, empathy, well not empathy, that's not right, but you know you click! You either click with somebody or you don't and there was something about her that meant, yeah, we didn't feel judged. And that was important. Because we respected her, then it made the process easier, I guess we felt more at ease. So I suppose experience means a lot to me really.

Sue – (Lily's partner) Yeah, in terms of her personal character, I thought she was bright, she was funny, it was professional as well. It wasn't like we were sitting chatting to a friend.

Lily – She never gave anything of herself away.

Sue – Never ever said a single thing to us about herself.

Barbara – She was warm, um, not afraid to ask things, not afraid to ask questions. I mean we were not afraid to respond either so it was pretty open.

Jenny – What I hear sometimes from other people about what their social workers asked that sometimes seemed inappropriate, or to show a certain level of ignorance about what it means to be lesbian, or what it means to come out to your parents, or all those kinds of things that – I mean I don't even know if she was straight or not, she wouldn't give much away about her own life, but we just felt that she was completely, quite neutral about everything, and just helpful.

Three participants were able to compare their experiences of being assessed twice by different social workers:

Lucy – She really was just enthusiastic, really friendly, just put you at ease, it didn't feel like you were being put under the microscope. She was very apologetic for having to ask all these questions. She was just lovely weren't she?

Isobel (Lucy's partner) – With (name of the other social worker) it was more like she'd got a script, and that was her questions that she'd got to ask, '… and they are the ones I'm asking.' It was like, 'I've got a tick box, tick, tick, tick. Right, I've done that.' And she forgot to be human in the process.

The majority of participants had attended panel. Participants all found this 'scary' and 'nerve-wracking', and 'a grilling':

Jenny – Well, it was telling that at one point, one of the panel members said, 'What is your Achilles heel then, because it (the assessment report) almost sounded like too good to be true?' There was also a question from the medical advisor who said, 'who will be the father figure or who will be the father figures in your life?', and I wasn't sure if he was like, meaning, 'which of us was going to be the father figure?' or 'who in your social network is going to be the father figure?', and we could see that the social workers and a lot of the panel members were sort of cringing at the word 'father figure' (Laughing) and I sort of gasped a bit at that, but luckily Nazma (Jenny's partner) was very good, and she said, 'Oh I suppose you mean, ' will there be male role models in the life of this child?' and went on by saying,'yes there will be, we don't live in a women only world, we've got brothers and fathers and male friends so….'

Lily – Oh initially it was quite scary. 'Cos there's a horseshoe table and zillions of people sitting there. And you know, they fire questions at you.

Sue – And lots of smiling I remember. It was very welcoming on that level, and I remember the questions being asked about our son's birth father. And what his relationship would be to any adopted child. I definitely remember that!

Participants' experience of matching was varied, with some people waiting a matter of weeks from being approved before being given details about their child, whilst others waited up to two years for the match with their child. In examining the reasons given by participants for this variation, there were no consistent themes. Some participants were immediately placed on the Adoption Register. Others were encouraged to be as proactive as possible in seeking a match via sources such as 'Be My Parent' and approaching other Local Authorities directly, and yet others were matched very quickly with children from their assessing agency who were waiting to be adopted. One couple had specifically requested that they be matched with a child with learning disabilities, which they were. Three couples had been explicitly told during their assessment (these had occurred in1997, 2006 and 2007) that they would not be matched with babies, because babies requiring adoption were rare and they would be placed with heterosexual parents. None of the participants explicitly said to the agency that they wanted to be matched with a baby. Two of these couples were then matched with children under 1 year of age.

Introductions between the adopter and the child seemed to be a 'can of worms', with the relationship between the adopters and the foster carers consistently the area of the interview where participants voiced the most difficulties.

> *Barbara* – Before we were to meet Mark, we went along to the foster carers and met them first, which was awful, they were something! I mean of the whole thing, that's the bit that sticks in my throat the most ... the foster carers. Um, we went along to meet her, not him, he was out at work, but I don't think he wanted to meet us anyway, just to find out a bit about Mark, and his routines and all the rest of it ... and at that stage and you could see she was just bristling, this woman, she really didn't like us, and she came up with some really strange things like, 'Mark loves bacon', as if she thought if he came to live with us he'd never have bacon, 'cos I think she'd assumed that we were vegetarian, because all lesbians are vegetarians, so we had all of that ... they just would not let him go, they didn't want to let him go, they tried to undermine every introduction they possibly could, it was a really stressful period.

Social workers did not appear to be significantly involved in the introductions, taking a back seat after the plans had been drawn up, and leaving the foster carers to facilitate the introductions and this was hugely problematic for the majority of participants. The introduction plans were subject to review midway through the introductory period, but by this stage most participants said they were desperate to get the introductions finished.

> *Sue* – It was quite hard work initially . We weren't offered a cup of tea or anything and nor were we offered any toys to play with. We would have to play for then ... hours ... in the living room with her shoe, because there wasn't a toy to play with. You know, and the telly would be on quite a lot wouldn't it? She (the foster carer) did exactly the minimum that was required. It was agony that week. Wasn't it?

> *Lily* – Yeah. Absolute agony.

How the adoption assessment was used by the prospective adopters:

The participants were generally positive about their experience of going through the adoption assessment and showed insight and understanding for the process as a whole.

> *Jacqui* – Because I don't think that any talking about anything can actually prepare you for doing it, um, it gets you to think about what's involved, gets you to just focus ... but until you're actually faced with it there and then, I don't think it can.

Susan (Jacqui's Partner) – I don't think anything can prepare you fully for, really for the reality of having the responsibility of a little person all of the time, it's the biggest responsibility you will ever, ever have in the whole of your life. And it's bloody difficult. And infuriating at times, so no, I don't think it can prepare you, but I think, how can I try and say, I think if you really weren't ready for it, it would knock you down, so I think when you do reach the end and you get approved, you are ready for the challenge that lies ahead, you're not perhaps prepared for it, but you're ready for it. Does that make sense?

A number of participants were already parents and the relationship between the assessment and the experience of caring for an adopted child was different for them.

Cecelia – The process I think was quite useful in flushing out the issues that we have and enabled us to arrive at a clarity and consensus about the type of child that we were able to parent and some of the issues that might emerge from parenting an adopted child. In hindsight I think nothing really prepared us for what we then experienced which was (pause) ... significantly different to what we'd expected and that was to do with assumptions about parenting, competence in parenting birth children, and thinking that parenting an adopted child who had been significantly damaged was going to be, well not easy, but I don't think we were prepared as we should have been for the difficulties and challenges that we then faced ... umm ... and I think we underestimated that.

Sue – I guess because we did have a birth child who had been fairly easy, you know, I think we had to pull together and dig deep in terms of our resources as a couple and as parents to get through some of the stuff ... like when I reached the, 'I can't deal with this' kind of times. And there were some real times for that first of six months or so, when I felt absolutely at breaking point.

However, overall, participants valued the assessment experience. For the majority it offered a structured preparation time – an opportunity to talk and reflect on what being a parent to an adopted child might involve, and the skills required to undertake this task competently and well. For most people, the level of intrusion into their private lives over a considerable period of time was bearable, justified by the enormity of the task they were about to undertake.

Lily – Whenever you see all these programmes on television about adoption you see obviously people's experiences with assessments which are 99% of the time presented as this dreadful kind of grilling or unfair. I didn't feel that. I felt it was really fair and you know, what was asked was totally reasonable to ask.

The assessing agency's approach to raising and discussing issues about sexuality and lesbianism:

Some social workers were able to integrate the sexuality of the adopters into the assessment that was undertaken. Other social workers completely avoided talking about it.

> *Cecelia* – The social worker who was assessing us had no issues with us being a lesbian couple at all, and that vindicated our choice in going to this local authority who were experienced and knowledgeable about assessing lesbians and gay couples for adoption, and I wouldn't make that assumption because it wasn't my experience in the second assessment that I went through, where it was evidently the first time she had assessed a lesbian couple.

> *Jacqui* – Well, they certainly asked about our background, of our previous relationships and coming out to our families and that. And the impact that it had had and, but it wasn't, I don't remember it being a huge issue, it was just discussed because it was a part of our lives. You know, the fact that we're now together and ....

> *Susan* (Jacqui's partner) – I think you were probably questioned on it more than me.

> *Jacqui* – Yeah. Because I'd been married to a man before.

Questions about the quality of people's relationships were asked by assessing social workers. Inquiries were made about people's 'coming out' stories, their relationships with their birth families, friendship networks, and integration into the local community. Whilst most of the assessments occurred without conflict emerging between the social worker and adopter regarding the relevance of certain questions, this was not always the case.

> *Lucy* – [the assessing social worker asked] 'If we were talking to someone for the first time on the phone and you were describing yourself, what would you say?' Well I'm 6 foot, I've got peroxide blonde dyed hair, blue eyes, white um, that's about it. She said, 'well wouldn't you say you were a lesbian?' No. Would you say you were heterosexual?

> (Laughter.)

> *Lucy* – If I don't know someone – that's none of their business! And she was like, 'well, I would say that I'm black.' Well you are black! Yeah, ok I'm gay, but I don't shout about my sexuality the first time I speak to someone, and that sort

of didn't get us off on a very good footing did it? She couldn't understand where I was coming from, and I'm sorry but I don't think that's anyone's business.

The 'male role model' question was asked of all participants except one.

> *Stella* – Definitely. Yes, we were asked the rote questions about role models, dealing with bullying and teasing in school.

> *Susan* – Just panel (asked) with regards to the male role model question, yeah, which is so predictable.

This still appears to be an issue for social workers and panel members. However some social workers explained to participants that they were raising this to pre-empt questions that panel might have asked.

> *Jenny* – And so, she never really enquired (about sexuality), she never enquired beyond the sort of 'male role model' thing, but in a sense she was also just making sure we put in the information that would be required.

How have things changed over the last ten years?

Many things have changed in the adoption field over the past ten years, most notably the legal framework, including: the Adoption and Children Act 2002, which enables lesbians and gay men in partnerships (not necessarily in civil partnerships) to jointly adopt, and for the partner of the birth parent of a child (or children) to apply to adopt as a step parent; and the Equality Act (Sexual Orientation) Regulations 2007, which prohibits discrimination on the grounds of sexual orientation in providing goods, facilities and services, and this includes adoption services. This means that social workers have a responsibility to ensure that the assessment service they offer prospective lesbian and gay adopters is commensurate to that provided to heterosexual applicants. It would appear from the experiences of the 11 participants in this study, some who were assessed after this change in legislation, that there is still a gap between what the law says should happen and what is occurring in practice, a point made by Dugmore and Cocker (2008) and Brown and Cocker (2008). Jenny's initial experience of the adoption agency telling her where she may encounter prejudice in the adoption process is, on the one hand, refreshingly honest, in that the social worker is being honest about the institutional homophobia that is present at all levels within the system. However, on the other hand, it is concerning because the issues raised are starkly similar to many of the points made by Hicks and McDermott (1999) in their research ten years ago. From this small study, for three participants to tell me that local authorities are still publically stating in 2006, 2007 and 2009 that lesbians and gay men will not automatically be considered for babies solely on the basis of their sexuality, is concerning (and illegal).

> *Susan* – The main thing they do wrong is part of the assessment, in respect of it being something that might even put you off even going through the assessment, is they say, ' you will not get a baby.' And they are still saying it now in 2009, they are still saying, 'you will not get a baby. If you are a lesbian or gay couple you won't get a baby. We will give a baby to a heterosexual couple.' Um, and that might actually put you off even stepping on that rung of the ladder to go towards assessment, and that's a bit scary I think.

> *Jacqui* – We have raised it with them a couple of times.

> *Susan* – We've argued this point with them quite often, because we believe it's wrong.

> *Jacqui* – If they say that, they should say that to everybody. Or not at all.

However there were many areas of good practice identified by participants. Some of the participants' social workers demonstrated in their practice a complexity to their thinking which easily incorporated sexuality into the adoption assessment process. Some social workers are able to ask about the 'coming out' experience of lesbian adopters, which is different to the experience of heterosexual carers, whilst others cannot do this – they are almost embarrassed to mention it, possibly so they are not accused of being homophobic, or possibly because they are on an educative journey themselves during the assessment process.

> *Cecelia* – the second social worker said quite openly at some point that she'd never assessed a family like us before, and was obviously struggling at the beginning to understand our family and how we worked ....

This may indicate a need for further training on this issue, with service user involvement, but as Dugmore and Cocker (2008) indicate, training is not the sole answer in changing people's views and attitudes to difference in family forms and structures. Interestingly, in terms of a continuing interest in raising standards and making a positive contribution to adoption beyond their immediate family, since successfully adopting children, three of the women I interviewed are now independent members of adoption panels, and seven of the eleven women had continuing roles in adoption preparation sessions within their assessing local authority.

There were two areas that emerged from this study where further research could clarify whether issues raised are specific to lesbian and gay applicants or apply to other applicants' experience of adoption. The first area relates to the ways in which prospective adopters view the adoption assessment process. There was consensus that it was useful but can never prepare you for what is to follow, and it may be that this finding is not related to sexuality but to adoption generally.

The second area is the adopters' experience of the role of foster carers in the introduction process. Hicks and McDermott (1999) also identified this issue. This might be to do with foster carers experiencing difficulties in 'letting go' of children because they have formed an attachment, rather than because of blatant homophobia. Some of the experiences of the participants of this study suggest that the homosexuality of adopters compounds an already emotionally charged situation. The support that foster carers receive during the introductory process may require further examination.

The role of the assessing social worker is important to consider as one of 'gatekeeper' for specific types of families being approved in this process. Adoption social workers are involved in assessing families seen as suitable for children in care where adoption has been agreed as a plan for their future. It is the child's social worker who is ultimately responsible for making a decision regarding the best family match for a child. Further understanding of the way in which these dynamics work is integral to understanding the subtle and not so subtle signs of the manifestations of heterosexism and homophobia within a large institutional process. Hicks' (2000) description of the social workers' key qualities of 'good lesbians' are reflected in the small sample of lesbians included in this study. This aside, the confidence of the group of women I interviewed in coming forward to engage critically and constructively with the adoption process and resulting systems is encouraging, because all have successfully navigated the difficult task of the 'state being in your sitting room' and this is no easy task. Brown and Cocker comment:

> Until recently, the private domestic homes of lesbians and gay men have been the only environment where they could express themselves and pursue their lives in an open manner, free from prejudicial scrutiny. Lesbians and gay men who have put themselves forward as carers and adopters have had to marry the public and the private, in terms of their homes and their private lives becoming subject to scrutiny by public agencies (Brown and Cocker 2008: 28).

This says something about the complexity of 'people's lives in the making' (Butler 2009) – where 'becoming' is a process that never ends or stops.

> *Barbara* – The assessment ... it captures something at that moment in time, doesn't it, for you, your family. By the time Mark arrived, you know, things were different again. Families are constantly changing aren't they?

Conclusion

This study has provided an opportunity to examine the adoption assessment experiences of a small number of lesbian adopters. Most of the participants reported experiences that were positive about most aspects of their adoption assessment, with many experienced social workers demonstrating a complexity to their thinking about sexuality, generally associated with good practice in this area.

However, whilst the quality of social work practice in this area may be at last showing tentative signs of change in terms of social work confidence and competence, it is clear there is still more work to do. There were a number of issues consistently raised about particular aspects of the assessment process that indicates some reluctance by social workers to change embedded practices or to understand the manifestations of prejudice and discrimination. This was evidenced through the continued use of the 'male role model' question being consistently asked in assessments. Additionally, some social workers did not want to appear homophobic in the way they raised certain issues with prospective adopters and this led to gaps in what was covered in the assessments about applicants' sexuality. As Brown and Cocker comment, 'the paradox is that to ignore this aspect of the human experience stands in stark contrast to the prurient fascination often focused upon lesbian and gay sex' (Brown and Cocker 2008:26).

Two additional areas were raised in this study regarding the experiences of prospective adopters after they are approved. Firstly, there is more work to do in ensuring equity in how matching occurs between children and prospective adopters, and this should centre on the paramountcy of the child. Secondly, there is further work that social workers and fostering link workers can do to support foster carers and adopters through the process of introductions. However, these findings may not apply solely to the experience of lesbian adopters – these are considerations for practice that could have wider benefits. Additional research comparing and contrasting the experience of lesbian adopters with the experiences of other adopters may assist in clarifying whether these areas are problematic for adopters regardless of their sexuality, ethnicity and family structure or whether there are subtle and not so subtle differences in the assessment experiences of lesbians and gay men that mean that their experiences of adoption are further compounded by their sexuality.

References

Bagilhole, B. 2009. *Understanding Equal Opportunities and Diversity: The social differentiations and intersections of inequality*. Bristol: Policy Press.

Barrett, H. & Tasker, F. 2001. Growing up with a Gay Parent: Views of 101 gay fathers on their sons' and daughters' experiences. *Educational and Child Psychology*, 18(1), 62–77.

Barrett, H. & Tasker, F. 2002. Gay Fathers and their children: what we know and what we need to know. *Lesbian and Gay Psychology Review*, 3, 3–10.

Brown, H.C. 1991. Competent child-focused practice: working with lesbian and gay carers. *Adoption and Fostering*, 15(2), 11–17.

Brown, H.C. 1998. Social Work and Sexuality: Working with Lesbians and Gay Men. Basingstoke: Macmillan.

Brown, H.C. 2008. Social Work and Sexuality, Working with Lesbians and Gay Men: What Remains the Same and What is Different? *Practice: Social Work in Action*, 20(4), 265–275.

Brown, H.C. & Cocker, C. 2008. Lesbian and gay fostering and adoption: out of the closet into the mainstream? *Adoption and Fostering*, 32(4) 19–30.

Brown, H.C. & Cocker, C. 2011. *Social Work with Lesbians and Gay Men*. London: Sage.

Brown, H.C. & Kershaw, S. 2008. The Legal Context for Social Work with Lesbians and Gay Men in the UK: Updating the Educational Context. *Social Work Education*, 27(2), 122–130.

Butler, J. 2009. *Frames of War: When is life Grievable?* London: Verso.

Cocker, C. & Anderson, J. 2011. *Adoption, in Advanced Social Work with Children and Families*, edited by C. Cocker & L. Allain. Exeter: Learning Matters.

Cocker, C. & Brown, H.C. 2010. Sex, Sexuality and Relationships: Developing Confidence and Discernment when Assessing Lesbian and Gay Prospective Adopters. *Adoption and Fostering*, 34(1), 20–32.

Cocker, C., and Hafford Letchfield, T. 2010. Critical Commentary: Out and Proud? Social Work's relationship with lesbians and gay men. *British Journal of Social Work*, 40(6). http://bjsw.oxfordjournals.org/cgi/content/abstract/bcp158v1 [accessed 20 March 2010].

Department of Children, Schools and Families. 2007. *Statistical First Release: Children Looked After in England (including adoption and care leavers) year ending 31st March 2007*. http://www.dcsf.gov.uk/rsgateway/DB/SFR/s000741/SFR27-2007rev.pdf [accessed 26 November 2009].

Department of Children, Schools and Families. 2008. *Statistical First Release: Children Looked After in England (including adoption and care leavers) year ending 31ˢᵗ March 2008*.http://www.dcsf.gov.uk/rsgateway/DB/SFR/s000810/SFR23-2008_Final.pdf [accessed 26 November 2009].

Department of Children, Schools and Families. 2009. *Statistical First Release: Children Looked After in England (including adoption and care leavers) year ending 31ˢᵗ March 2009*. http://www.dcsf.gov.uk/rsgateway/DB/SFR/s000878/SFR25-2009Version2.pdf [accessed 26th November 2009].

Department for Education and Skills. 2006. *Preparing and Assessing Prospective Adopters*. London: DFES.

Department of Health. 2003. *Adoption: National Minimum Standards*. London: The Stationery Office.

Dugmore, P. & Cocker, C. 2008. Legal, Social and Attitudinal Changes: An Exploration of Lesbian and Gay Issues in a Training Programme for Social Workers in Fostering and Adoption. *Social Work Education*, 27(2),159–168.

Erich, S. 2005. Gay and Lesbian Adoptive Families: An Exploratory Study of Family Functioning, Adoptive Child's Behaviour and Familial Support Networks. *Journal of Family Social Work*, 9(1), 17–32.

Erich, S., Kanenberg, H., Case, K., Allen, T. & Bogdanos, T. 2009. An empirical Analysis of factors affecting adolescent attachment in adoptive families with homosexual and straight parents. *Children and Youth Services Review*, 31(3), 398–404.

Fish, J. 2007. Getting equal: The implications of new regulations to prohibit sexual orientation discrimination for health and Social Care. *Diversity in Health and Social Care*, 4, 221–228.

Fostering Network. 2006. *Improving Effectiveness in Foster Care Recruitment.* London: Fostering Network.

Golombok, S., Spencer, A. & Rutter, M. 1983. Children in lesbian and single parent households: Psychosexual and psychiatric appraisal. *Journal of Child Psychology and Psychiatry*, 24, 551–572.

Golombok, S. 2000. *Parenting: what really counts?* London: Routledge.

Hicks, S. 1993. T*he Expereinces of Lesbians and Gay Men in Fostering and Adoption: A Study of the Impact of the Process of Assessment upon Prospective Carers. Economic and Social Science*, University of Manchester: MA Thesis.

Hicks, S. 1996. The 'last resort'?: lesbian and gay experiences of the social work assessment process in fostering and adoption. *Practice*, 8(2), 15–24.

Hicks, S. 1997. Taking the risk? Assessing lesbian and gay carers, in *Good Practice in Risk Assessment and Risk Management 2: Protection, rights and responsibilities*, edited by H. Kemshall & J. Pritchard. London: Jessica Kingsley Publishers.

Hicks, S. 1998. *Familiar Fears: The assessment of lesbian and gay fostering and adoption applicants.* Applied Social Science, Lancaster University: PhD thesis.

Hicks, S. 2000. Good lesbian, bad lesbian … regulating heterosexuality in fostering and adoption assessments. *Child & Family Social Work*, 5(2), 157–68.

Hicks, S. 2005a. Lesbian and gay foster care and adoption: a brief UK history. *Adoption & Fostering,* 29(3), 42–56.

Hicks, S. 2005b. Queer genealogies: tales of conformity and rebellion amongst lesbian and gay foster carers and adopters. *Qualitative Social Work*, 4(3), 293–308

Hicks, S. 2008. Thinking through sexuality. *Journal of Social Work*, 8(1), 65–82.

Hicks, S. with Greaves, D. 2007. *Practice Guidance on Assessing Gay and Lesbian Foster Care and Adoption Applicants.* Manchester: Manchester City Council.

Hicks, S. & McDermott, J. (eds) 1999. *Lesbian and Gay Fostering and Adoption: Extraordinary Yet Ordinary.* London: Jessica Kingsley.

Hill, N. 2009. *The Pink Guide to Adoption for Lesbians and Gay Men.* London: BAAF.

Hudson, W. & Ricketts, W. 1980. A strategy for the measurement of Homophobia. *Journal of Homosexuality*, 5(4), 357–372.

Kindle, P.A. & Erich, S. 2005. Perceptions of social support among heterosexual and homosexual adopters. *Families in Society*, 86(4), 541–546.

Leung, P., Erich, S. & Kanenberg, H. 2005. A comparison of family functioning in gay/lesbian, heterosexual and special needs adoptions. *Children and Youth Services Review*, 27(9), 1031–1044.

Logan, J. & Sellick, C. 2007. Lesbian and Gay Fostering and Adoption in the United Kingdom: Prejudice, Progress and the Challenges of the Present. *Social Work and Social Sciences Review*, 13(2), 35–47.

Lord, J (2008) *The Adoption Process in England: A Guide for Children's Social Workers*. London: BAAF.

Mallon, G. 2007. Assessing Lesbian and Gay prospective foster and adoptive families: A Focus on the Home Study process. *Child Welfare*, 86(2), 67–86.

Mallon, G. & Betts, B. 2005. *Recruiting, Assessing and Supporting Lesbian and Gay Carers and Adopters*. London: BAAF.

Patterson, C.J. 2004. Gay fathers, in *The Role of the Father in Child Development*, Fourth Edition, edited by M.E. Lamb. New York: John Wiley.

Patterson, C.J. 2005. *Lesbian and Gay Parenting*. Washington DC: American Psychological Association.

Ryan, S. & Whitlock, C. 2009. Becoming Parents: Lesbian Mothers' Adoption Experience, in *Social Work with Lesbian Parent Families: Ecological Perspectives*, edited by Lucy R. Mercier & Rena D. Harold, New York: Routledge.

Skeates, J. & Jabri, D. (eds) 1988. *Fostering and Adoption by Lesbians and Gay Men*. London Strategic Policy Unit: London.

Stott, A. 2009. Adoption Register Overview: Experience of the Adoption Register regarding lesbian and gay adopters. *Sharing Evidence, Overcoming Resistance – Celebrating the Role of Lesbian and Gay Carers*, BAAF Conference 11th May 2009: London.

Tasker, F. 1999. Children in Lesbian-led families: a review. Clinical Child *Psychology and Psychiatry*, 4(2), 153–166.

Tasker, F. 2005. Lesbian Mothers, Gay Father and their children: A Review. *Journal of Developmental and Behavioural Pediatrics*, 26, 224–240.

Tasker, F. and Golombok, S. 1991. Children raised by Lesbian Mothers: The Empirical Evidence. *Family Law*, 21, 184–187.

Chapter 10

Identity, Emotion Work and Reflective Practice: Dealing with Sexuality, Race and Religion in the Classroom

Cathy Aymer and Rachana Patni

Introduction

This chapter focuses on two related questions that emerged spontaneously from our practice as social work educators. The widening participation agenda in higher education in general and in some social work courses in particular has led to an increasingly diverse student population in many areas of the country. Whilst we herald this development, we recognize that in a diverse classroom, there are various voices and the interaction between these voices can often raise questions that are relevant to understanding issues of social justice and social inclusion. The diversity in the classroom cannot just be viewed from the perspective of the student but also from that of the lecturer, for there is now a growing number of minority ethnic academics, like ourselves, whose voices may also be different from that of the mainstream. So we set out with these naïve inquiries:

- How do we understand and manage interactions in a diverse classroom?
- How can we improve the quality of our pedagogical practices in the light of this?

These are both ontological and methodological questions, which would be difficult to address without linking them to identity (both personal and professional). These questions are particularly pertinent ones in a value-laden profession such as social work. It follows that in social work education; we are also engaged in a value-laden education. When professional attitudes are breached in the classroom, it might call for individual and institutional change. We are interested in questions of social justice and social inclusion and part of our identity comes from this value-committed stance. As educators we have to start by making explicit our value commitments and owning our multi-faceted identities because we maintain our engagement with our value-based professional field.

The task of preparing social work students for professional practice is fraught with dilemmas, with which we struggle. One such dilemma is that we are engaged in creating social workers who are able to critically work toward social change, while also being able to be responsive to the creeping managerialism (Burton and Broek 2008) that is part and parcel of contemporary welfare delivery. Another dilemma is that of teaching empathy and non-judgemental attitudes when these ideas might imply a revisiting of the students' entire 'selfhood'. In dealing with these dilemmas, we start from a position that professional knowledge is not only for the acquisition of information, what Paulo Freire calls the banking system of education, but that it is about transforming minds, beings and knowledge itself. Freire was very clear that learning could be liberatory (Freire 1972) and points out that knowledge has been developed and internalized to develop 'cultures of silence' of the oppressed. Our commitment to transformation requires the un-silencing of oppressed perspectives.

Stating the problem

For some years we have observed a certain dynamic unfolding in our classrooms. Following the anti-racist and anti-sexist debates of the 1980s and anti-oppressive and anti-discriminatory agendas in social work education, we now have a diverse student body as well as a diverse group of academic staff. This leads to a classroom in which some identities are more visible than others. For example, in our case, black women are the visible majority, while gay men and lesbians, both black and white, remain invisible. With some black students, there is often an outspoken religiosity and an acceptance of fundamentalist beliefs. It would not be an overstatement to say that the most fundamentally religious are often the black students. It should not be forgotten that some white students are religious fundamentalists as well, but they tend not to be as outspoken. When we speak about this we apply this not only to Christians but also to some Muslims (we have not observed this tendency with other faiths). This outspoken religiosity can bring a very oppressive and homophobic climate into the classroom. This is not surprising given that the classroom reflects the real world, where, at present, there is a possible split within the Anglican Communion since in all recent debates many African churches/bishops have been outspokenly homophobic. This is echoed in other denominations, where, for example, the Pope is reported to be mounting a challenge against equality legislation in the UK for fear that the Catholic Church may be 'forced' to ordain gay clergy (Butt 2010).

In particular, in this chapter, we focus on what happens when black women make oppressive comments in classroom discussions. The response is often, initially, one of silence. Being much immersed in church work and a church community, they feel 'empowered' to voice their homophobic and discriminatory opinions. After all they can claim that this is backed up by scripture and religious doctrine. There are several outcomes from such 'outbursts', two of which we highlight here. One result is that challenging these comments can be interpreted as racist in their impact, as these black women feel attacked for voicing their views and feel that such challenges carry racist undertones. Another is that it becomes the 'burden' of white men to 'come out' in this most intolerant atmosphere. Therefore, as lecturers, we find ourselves having to ask these questions:

- How do we engage with this kind of an audience?
- Can students really pick and choose which groups they can legitimately discriminate against?
- How do we make other students feel comfortable enough to challenge this?

Hicks (2008) has drawn attention to how sexuality is theorized within social work. Others have spoken of a forced heterosexuality (Myers 2008) and we observe gay and lesbian students having to 'pass' as heterosexual. In the classroom we are dealing with an everyday heterosexism that impacts on students' social values, their sense of morality and their views about normative sexual and gender identities. We have to challenge ourselves and our students in order to help them question their adherence to heteronormativity and begin to become inclusive of gay sexuality.

In conceptualizing and intensifying this challenge, we have to first state our position as straight women who feel that we must interrogate heteronormativity, because we are all implicated in its (re)production. While we do not wish to essentialize a 'dialectic relationship between lesbian and straight women' (Jeyasingham 2008:4), we acknowledge that in a classroom context we are more likely to be perceived as 'straight' women with heterosexual commitments. In owning this standpoint we wonder whether the experiences of those lecturers who are out as gay or lesbian find the classroom a hostile environment, or whether they find these issues any easier to handle than we do. Even when we subscribe to post structural conceptualizations of our identities, we often have to adopt a position of strategic essentialism in order to foreground certain marginal identities and seek material transformations. Therefore our task is about engaging in an analysis of sexuality, race and gender in the classroom without essentializing any of these concepts.

Why is this problematic for us?

A commitment to anti-discriminatory practice in social work interventions is at the heart of our trouble with this situation. As black educators we feel the frustration of witnessing black women reinforce racial stereotypes and failing to make the link between racial oppression and the oppression of other minorities. The pain of black gay and lesbian students who have been fearful of other black students also wounds us. They have to 'pass' as heterosexuals because they risk too much if they come out in the hostile atmosphere of the classroom. So too do white lesbians. A multi-cultural and diverse existence always involves dealing with differences positively and we struggled with how best to achieve this in a classroom context.

Fish (2008) has identified many of the taken-for-granted assumptions about gay life and we hear these in the classroom. Others have looked at the ways in which students and academics view issues of heterosexism and homophobia (Ben-Ari 2001 and Foreman and Quinlan 2008). Brown and Kershaw (2008) have drawn attention to the legal context for lesbians and gay men. We are, however, concerned about our students' practice with lesbian, gay, bisexual and transgendered (LGBT) service users and with their colleagues. For example, how are these students going to work with a young person with an emerging gay or lesbian or questioning their sexuality? We are also committed to enabling an enquiry about how heternormativity structures our lives, by "policing" (Jeyasingham 2008:13) our "desires and behaviours and interactions" (Jeyasingham 2008:13), thereby not deluding ourselves that heteronormativity is something that only homosexuals struggle with.

We also observe how the students still operate with an idealized model of the family and this exists as the family in their mind. The paradox is that many of these students have been reared in single mother households or in extended families and are now rearing their own children in single mother households. They seem unable to make the links between how their own families have been stereotyped and how they reproduce these stereotypes when they speak of LGBT families. They are not able to realize that the processes which maintain discrimination and oppression take similar forms across all social divisions. Our aim is to enable students to make links with all other aspects of inclusion and exclusion, and comprehend the similarities between the Othering of 'gay sexuality' and the Othering of all other identities. We know how in post-colonial societies, sexual identity is racialized and racial identity is sexualized, and how black heterosexuality can often be fetishized. We have seen how a spurious equation has been made between HIV/AIDS and gay sexuality in the general population and know that social work students are not immune from common social discourses.

Without the recognition of the shared processes and impact of different types of marginalization by the student group, we have to deal with uncomfortable topics in the classroom that come from an unreflective space. As professional educators we are engaged in the process of secondary socialization where we ask students to question and, perhaps, to move away from their primary socialized values and adopt professional values. Our attempts at secondary socialization are often limited in their immediate impact because these students believe that they have a right to these discriminatory attitudes and values and their question to us is: who are we to re-socialize them? This produces an implicit resistance in the students.

Emotion work

The effort we put into this type of teaching, and in moving beyond this resistance, means that we have to do emotion work (Hochschild 1983). Emotion work focuses on the acts of individuals within organizations that help them present the required emotional persona in organizational contexts and is a larger set of activities rather than the mere presentation of desirable emotions of organizational gain. In order to understand emotion work and the related concept of emotion management (Bolton 2001) we need to first comprehend the idea of feeling rules. Feeling rules are informed by ideological aspects and are like other sorts of rules because they delineate zones within which certain feelings become permissible or are deemed appropriate. Management of feelings could be an outcome of responding to issues such as legitimacy and conformity, and therefore feelings could be managed in response to significantly varied rules (Bolton 2004). Hence, feeling rules are social guidelines that enable us to determine what normal emotion in different contexts is. A typology of feeling rules has been developed by Bolton and Boyd (2003), where they propose that feeling rules could be organizationally prescribed, determined by professional codes, by social norms or by the ideal of caring. These then lead to different forms of emotion management, namely pecuniary, prescriptive, presentational or philanthropic.

Emotion management is the type of work it takes to cope with feeling rules and continue to present ourselves as 'normal'. We propose that part of the problem we have to cope with is that our emotion management has to incorporate juggling between different feeling rules – between prescriptive and philanthropic feeling rules, but also between prescriptive and pecuniary feeling rules. This juggling requires continuous reflection and performance of different aspects of our professional commitments, namely, those of being educators, and those of being social workers. Much of this emotion work is that we have to hold back an aspect of our self in order to allow students to make their transformational journeys. We have to do this in order to get them to reflect and make connections so that they are able to learn and develop. The main question we have to answer is: why do we need to transform them? To answer this we need to undertake political theorizing, making connections to service user perspectives, feminist perspectives and postcolonial understandings.

In this way we can demonstrate to students that this learning is not just an instrumental response, but a subjective one that connects epistemology and ontology. To do this as educators, we need to conceptualize our pedagogic practice in the classroom as emotion work, and in doing so we are looking for ways of improving the quality of that practice. However, this transformational input is not unproblematic; neither is the continued holding back of particular aspects of our selves. We recognize that we have to breach our own values from time to time, i.e. instead of enabling students to emerge with the ideas, sometimes we may have to seek to impose professional attitudes. It is the dilemma of social work education that even if we have a radical agenda in relation to anti discriminatory practice, we are educating students to become part of a normative profession and we need to explore the tensions inherent in this and it makes the conceptualization as emotion work a very apt one.

This can be seen as the primary requirement to perform the role of a lecturer when dealing with race, religion and sexuality in the classroom. We also conceptualize value-based education as emotion work. When issues of sexuality emerge in classroom discussions they can be daunting, and many lecturers would prefer to 'let it go' especially if they deal with questions of identity. In order to deal with this fear, to prevent its immobilizing potential, we need to engage in reflective practice that provides us with strategies that move us forward in our secondary socialization efforts. We see the need to construct dialogical relationships with colleagues and with students and discover ways in which these can be beneficial to practice. We work more and more in research-led universities but it is incumbent on us as professional educators to keep in mind the dilemmas encountered in teaching. If we are to develop our pedagogical practices, we need to engage in supportive peer relationships and share our experiences; this is another kind of emotion work.

Value laden education such as social work education also lends itself to pluralistic voices, and the interactive or elaborated pedagogical style (Murray and Aymer 2008) encourages student participation. This does not conceptualize students as 'ignorant people' who need to be taught, but as 'knowers' who need to be engaged in another conceptual area. This is different from disciplines that identify themselves as purely scientific (thereby also claiming to be factual, objective and with singular truths). These types of classrooms, because of the diversity, the value base and the pedagogical approach, involve emotion work from the lecturer and this needs to be recognized as a common rather than an uncommon occurrence in professional education.

In linking emotion work to our work roles, we became interested in the concept of the tempered radical as developed by Meyerson (2001). She describes tempered radicals as people who want to succeed in their organizations, yet want to live by their values and identities. This is in a context where they are somehow at odds with the dominant culture of their organizations. Tempered radicals want to fit in and they want to retain what makes them different. They want to rock the boat, and they want to stay in it. (Meyerson 2001:xi). They engage in small local battles rather than wage dramatic wars, at times operating so quietly that they may not surface on the cultural radar as rebels or change agents. Sometimes they pave alternative roads just by quietly speaking up for their own personal truths or by refusing to silence aspects of themselves. Not heroic leaders of revolutionary change, rather they are cautious and committed catalysts who keep going and who slowly make a difference.

Meyerson goes on to describe the many ways that tempered radicals can make a difference. They range from resisting quietly and staying true to themselves at one end of the scale to organizing collective action at the other end. This links in with our findings that as black professionals we are consistently conscious of the ways in which our racial identities can make us outsiders within our university contexts.

We have a nuanced understanding of how we and other black lecturers have to withstand the dominant culture's definition of us and become steadfast in our own definition of self. The emotion work needed to hold on to our values that are often contradicted in practice can be a very draining experience. When so much energy has to be expended in defending ourselves against threats to our identity, we struggle to find the optimal level of emotional engagement. This can seem like dangerous space to occupy and so sometimes it can be easier to not discuss identities at all and at other times we can get completely consumed. This nuanced understanding helps us reflect on the parallels between working with issues of race and issues of sexuality in the classroom. Therefore the emotion work and the energy required in being a 'tempered' radical are felt in our role as educators in other scenarios as well. Both require a performance that is an outcome of emotional reflection.

In the light of the above reflective practice we constantly pose questions for ourselves, such as:

- How can we hold values and live them even if this makes us exposed and vulnerable?
- How can we continue to develop our self-reflective practices and continue to work with students in a sensitive manner that challenges the dominant discourses about sexuality, race and religion?
- What are the influences that one individual educator can have, and how can we demonstrate the influences we have had? How have we made a difference?
- How can we both inhabit our world-view and look through it at the same time? This is what we are inviting students to do when we challenge their discriminatory comments.

An example of how we have engaged in this type of reflection is that we allocate time to reflect together, take opposing positions in the discourse, and help the other person to think, become a devil's advocate and imagine different scenarios.

When working with students we have learnt to become skilled at setting ground rules about behaviour that is acceptable. We have learnt to demonstrate and model that it is OK to disagree: in doing this we demonstrate the difference between disagreement and hostility, how to hold ideas with passion and yet hold them with a lightness that enables us to take account of the Other. It has been important for us to understand that some present disagreements are the result of historical encounters and we need to be sensitive to these histories (see Patni 2007). Importantly, we have learnt to both use the silence effectively as well as show how it is possible to break this silence.

Telling the story and forming strategic interventions

When we started this reflective process, Rachana was a newly appointed lecturer and Cathy was a lecturer of some years' experience. However we had independently observed and were concerned about the same phenomenon (Aymer 1999), which occurred when issues of sexuality were being discussed, and the way that this has been intensified over the years. There were two ways in which we could have dealt with this: either by ignoring it because of the perceived fear of dealing with uncomfortable subjects, or by engaging with this as an inquiry which would take the form of reflective practice combined with theoretical conceptualizations. To enhance our development in this area, we engaged in action/reflection cycles (Reason 1994). In the reflection stage we explored theoretical positions and planned activities. In the action phase we tried these out in the classroom and then followed up with further reflection. The art was a constant engagement in the cyclical and iterative process.

It is in this context that we have come to engage with our students and to discuss this strange meeting, the intersectionality between race, religion and sexuality in the classroom. We have had to find different ways to use knowledge to make sense of these situations and help students to understand them. We have tried out different theoretical frameworks for understanding both the student world views and the lecturers engaging in emotion work. We have set out to find theoretical explanations at both the macro and the micro levels of analysis. Below we present two significant theoretical considerations, one that involves us rethinking religiosity and second that helped us think about how to 'be' in the classroom.

Understanding and rethinking religiosity

One interesting aspect that we have explored is that religion has been the positive force for survival for many black students. In the conundrums of today, religion has also been an organizing form that has helped them in their struggle by instilling in them a very palpable sense of faith, which serves them well and makes them keep going against adversity. However, those that are most resistant to change may have reasons and it is important to ascertain what these might be. One noteworthy consideration is that there might be a historical dimension. We have both observed and surmised that it is mostly neo-converts who most vociferously articulate the fundamentalist black Christian position. This might be telling us the story that the newly converted need to protect their identity, and in order to do this they need to phase out all doubts. They cannot tolerate challenges to their concepts because these are relatively newly acquired and must be fortified and defended at all costs. It is these fundamentals that are dear to their identity. Moreover, religious identity may have been very important in granting them the kind of life that they are grateful for because the strengths of the religion and its impact can sometimes be absolutely transformational. After all, religion may serve to provide them with a template that helps them to survive and as such has great adaptive potential.

However, the same template and the same orientation to religion can become maladaptive with respect to their ability to empathize with other human beings and to see other kinds of oppression. It is important here to distinguish between intrinsic and extrinsic attitudes toward religion and how these connect with prejudice. Allport (1979) suggested that for people who use religion as a means to communal ends, it can lead to prejudice but those that see religion as an end in itself are more likely to be more accepting of humanity. What is clear is that we are in a world where creationism and post-modernism are both visible forces because 'reason above religiosity' may have been a dictum of the Enlightenment but is not necessarily operational in all cases today.

Theoretical considerations

One of the ways in which we made sense of what was happening in the classroom was to reflect on different ways of understanding 'Me–Other' representations'. To do this we looked at different ways of viewing the world. In the first instance we looked at the world from the point of view of Aristotelian logic and in particular the Law of the excluded middle, which states that a thing is either one thing or another. We could see how this has produced 'either/or' logic which can leave us stuck in particular positions. The nature of oppression and discrimination is such that people cannot position themselves in both groups, i.e. they cannot see themselves as oppressive, even when they are being blatantly so, when their primary way of conceptualizing themselves is as the oppressed. This leads to an 'Either–Or' orientation to belongingness in a way that leads to certain conclusions, e.g. if you are black then you cannot also be homosexual. This also leads to the perpetuation of racial stereotypes and the vocal members with the dominant stories become the ones who are able to decide where other people should belong.

Secondly, we thought about Hegelian/Dialogic ways of viewing the world and lead to 'Both/And Logic', the ability to hold the one and the many together. This leads to a more inquiring, and therefore inclusive, way of viewing the relationship between Me and the Other. There is yet another possible world view, that of Vedanta – where both me and other are seen as embodiments of divinity and therefore are seen as sharing divinity; the difference between self and other is seen as an unhelpful illusion that needs to be challenged. Further, true human nature is seen as 'divine' (a layperson's guide can be found at http://www.vivekananda.org/faqs.asp). This stresses the oneness of the universe and shared existence and consciousness.

We observe that in these different ways of conceptualizing 'Me–Other' relationships that the "dichotomous oppositional differences" (Hill Colllins, 2004:110) which inform our understanding of the world needs to be challenged from a feminist perspective of distrust of binaries. We can see how a narrative approach towards people, thinking about identities in particular ways, can be useful here. After all, we have narratives about the self and the Other. How do we build an ontological approach in the classroom which can allow different narratives to co-exist? Usually, the self is privileged and the other is cast down. We hear our students putting forward stories that represent the 'dominant' stories of their culture or religion. There are religious stories, political stories, and all sorts of stories. What is most striking is that sometimes people can tell the same negative story about another group that has been used to oppress them. It is particularly poignant to hear black students using the exact language of prejudice and stereotype that has been used to oppress black people, and somehow they cannot make the connection. There are times when we have tried to show how this happens by saying to students, 'let us replace the word gay with the word black in what you have just said'. However the students often can respond with another story, namely, ' you can CHOOSE to be gay but you cannot choose to be black'. The important point here is that they credit a sense of agency (but see Hegarty 2002 for the opposite argument) in having a gay identity and therefore blame can follow. This then legitimizes their oppressive attitudes. Instead of allowing our students to hold on to their 'solid' selves that are mired in binaries and are resistant to change, we have to enable a transformation in their understanding of their selfhood as a post structural project that can change, and continue to become through engagement in certain performances.

How can change happen?

The major difficulty that lecturers face is how to change these 'Me–Other' representations. We could either strengthen opposing representations or weaken/ change existing ones. Representations can be seen not just as emanating from the media but also as the active outcome of everyday talk and the general discourse that represents certain groups of people. Within the classroom, change may not happen immediately but the disruptions caused by challenging of assumptions could create a reflective space where change could be meaningfully negotiated. We have used certain theoretical ways of understanding 'self' and 'other' to come up with ways in which comfort with discriminatory attitudes can be usefully disrupted. This understanding has helped in creating some classroom exercises that we use to disrupt the comfort with discrimination. We will turn later to discussing how our application of theoretical conversations led to the creation of a classroom exercise that caused a successful disruption of normative ideas.

Theory into action

We set out to find theoretical explanations at both macro and micro levels of analysis. The tasks that we engage in with students involve deconstructing of their dominant narratives and helping them to construct their worlds in a more inclusive manner. The challenge is to help them to understand that these dominant narratives are damaging to the self and to the Other. The social work classroom provides an opportunity for co–constructing with the Other. In order to do this, there are some key notions that can be used, such as, the difference between belief and knowledge; building social capital in the classroom; problematizing the concepts of empathy and of normality

Linking the notion of self to the concept of empathy

This is linked with identity and how people construct their identity as being only one thing. If they hold a unilinear view of identity then it's difficult for them to construct an identity which is multi-faceted. One might expect that empathy would be the outcome of being oppressed. In fact the complexity of oppression stems from the interconnection and overlap of social differences (Clifford and Burke 2007). Empathy is important wherever there is diversity so for example, whether we talk about class and caste in India or we talk about race and sexuality in the UK. The diverse classroom does not engender necessarily the right kind of space to enable people to share their views and develop an inter-subjectively shared world that overrides social differences.

Existence of difference can lead to dialogue but the same existence of difference can also lead to the exercise of unequal power. Dialogue is linked with Freire's notion of participation, conscientization and social change and also with reflexivity. It is therefore important to engage in dialogue and this can only happen if we get to know different people on a human basis. Undertaking this, will lead to building of social capital but, as is acknowledged by Clifford and Burke, it will be emotionally as well as intellectually difficult and will require time. Building bridges always does!

Case study – Florence

It is not always possible to create and facilitate a safe learning environment but we have recognized that it is possible to create a productive one. The following case study demonstrates how this was possible in one instance.[1]

Florence is a first year student on the MA in Social Work programme. She is a young black woman of African descent. Very early in the course she expressed some negative views about gay people, which she was clear to describe as coming from her strong Christian faith. In discussion with the other students she was respectful in listening to other views but was adamant about her entitlement to her views and that she had no intention of changing them. She was certain that she would never discriminate against gay or lesbian service users because she was able to separate her professional views from her personal views. I challenged her, and other students, quite hard in the classroom, but she stuck to her guns. She undertook a task which asked her to think about the world from the position of a

---

1   This example draws upon Cathy Aymer's experience and is therefore written in the first person.

gay man or lesbian, and she was again respectful in undertaking the exercise but did not seem willing to reflect beyond her belief system.

I did not see Florence again until much later in the academic year, on the day of the assessed presentations to the group. I was one of the assessors. The students were asked to present an issue from their practice placements. When it was Florence's turn, she explained that she had been placed in an organization and her practice was with LGBT young people. Not only did she describe the 'issue' but she also presented her journey of learning from the start of the course and how she had come to question her taken-for-granted assumptions and beliefs about heterosexuality and homosexuality.

After the presentation she sought me out for a private conversation and told me how angry she had been with me at the start for confronting her about her religious beliefs. In addition she had then hated me because she thought that I must have conspired to make sure she was sent to that particular placement in an LGBT agency. However, she was now really pleased that that this had happened because she had received the best learning experience of her life. Her faith was still as strong as ever but she had begun to understand that as a reflective practitioner you had to be prepared to open up and question your taken-for-granted assumptions. She had come to a fuller understanding of how her attitudes could be detrimental to her ability to work with these young people. I reassured her that I had had no involvement in finding her a placement; nor did I have the power in ordering the world so that students are placed in particular organizations. I expressed my pleasure that her experience had been such a positive one.

We are not claiming that the student was transformed by her interactions with us, but we can claim that as committed social work educators, it is our role to disrupt dominant discourses about sexuality. In so doing, we set the stage for discomfort and even anger about sensitive subjects because we recognize that learning can come about from this anger, discomfort and fear. This student did not wish to have any doubts about her Christian world view, so she was resistant to exploring her beliefs about the Other. She was willing to construct a conspiracy theory in order to categorize her experience and prevent disruption of her cognitive consonance. In reality she, over time, and opening up to new thinking, was able to broaden her horizons and extend her world view without losing herself. We are helping students to 'unlearn', not that their world view is wrong, but that they need not be limited by their world views in such a way that they do not see the Other or make links with the oppression of others.

It also shows that this journey, once begun in the classroom, can be completed anywhere and over any time period. We are involved in preparing the ground for a potential development that does not necessarily happen in the classroom, but can do so at any time during their professional lives.

Conclusion

We are convinced that challenging our own religions and cultures should be part and parcel of social work education. In doing this work we raise the more general question about the nature of a professional identity and how is it acquired. We have shown how we struggle daily with a variety of issues linked to sexuality, belief, knowledge and practice and how in doing so we are engaged in emotion work. We are also aware of the emotion work that our students will be expected to perform in their professional roles. Because of our value-committed stance, we are clear that leaving these issues unattended is not an acceptable way forward for professional educators. We have highlighted the need to start with challenging the self (both for students and lecturers), and have stressed the need for reflection that must be self/other oriented. We have seen the need to utilize different theoretical arguments as a means of embracing difference and challenging oppressive structures. The important aspect is the creation of the possibility of reflection, which could either be co-created or 'thrust' upon us, but this reflection is the only space for deconstructing the damaging effects that heteronormativity inflicts upon us through controlling our desires and limiting our empathic abilities.

References

Allport, G.W. 1979. *The Nature of Prejudice*. Reading, MA: Addison-Wesley.

Aymer, C. 1999. Teaching and Learning Anti-racist and Anti-discriminatory Practice, edited by R. Pierce & J. Weinstein, *Innovative Education and Training for Care Professionals*. London: Jessica Kingsley, 121–136.

Ben-Ari, A. 2001. Homosexuality and Heterosexism: Views from Academics in Helping Professions. *British Journal of Social Work*, 31(1), 119–123.

Bolton, S. & Boyd, C. 2003. Trolley Dolly or Skilled Emotion Manager? Moving on from Hochschild's Managed Heart. *Work, Employment & Society*, 17(2), 289–308.

Bolton, S. 2001. Changing faces: nurses as emotional jugglers. *Sociology of Health & Illness*, 23(1), 85–100.

Bolton, S. 2004. *Emotion Management in the Workplace*. Basingstoke: Palgrave Macmillan.

Brown, H.C. & Kershaw, S. 2008. The Legal Context for Social Work with Lesbians and Gay Men in the UK: Updating the Educational Context. *Social Work Education*, 27(2), 122–130.

Burton, J. & Broek, D. 2008. Accountable and Countable: Information Management Systems and the Bureaucratization of Social Work. *The British Journal of Social Work*, 1–17.

Butt, R. 2010.Your equality laws are unjust, pope tells UK before visit. *The Guardian*. 2 February 2010. http://www.guardian.co.uk/world/2010/feb/02/equality-laws-unjust-pope-uk [accessed 25 March 2010].

Clifford, D. & Burke, B. 2005. Developing Anti-oppressive ethics in the new curriculum. *Social Work Education*, 24(6), 677–692.

Fish, J. 2008. Far from Mundane: Theorising Heterosexism for Social Work Education. *Social Work Education*, 27(2), 182–193.

Foreman, M. & Quinlan, M. 2008. Increasing Social Work Students' Awareness of Heterosexism and Homophobia – A Partnership between a Community Gay Health Project and a School of Social Work. *Social Work Education*, 27(2), 152–158.

Freire, P. (1972) *Pedagogy of the Oppressed*. UK, Penguin.

Hegarty, P. 2002. 'It's not a choice, it's the way we're built': Symbolic Beliefs about Sexual Orientation in the US and Britain. *Journal of Community & Applied Social Psychology*, 12(3), 153–166.

Hicks, S. 2008. Thinking through Sexuality. *Journal of Social Work*, 8(1), 65–82.

Hill-Collins, P. 2004. Learning from the outsider within: the sociological significance of black thought. Edited by S.G. Harding, *The Feminist Standpoint Theory Reader: Intellectual and Political Controversies*. London: Routledge, 103–126.

Hochschild, A.R. 1983. *The Managed Heart: Commercialization of Human Feeling*. Berkeley: University of California Press.

Jeyasingham, D. 2008. Knowledge/Ignorance and the Construction of Sexuality in Social Work Education. *Social Work Education*, 27(2), 138–151.

Meyerson, D. 2001. *Tempered Radicals: How People Use Difference to Inspire Change at Work*. Boston, MA: Harvard Business School Press.

Murray, J. & Aymer, C. 2008. The Apparent Conflict between Commitment to the development of the Profession and the Imperatives of the Academy. *Social Work Education*, 28(1), 81–95.

Myers, S. 2008. Revisiting Lancaster: More Things that Every Social Work Student Should Know. *Social Work Education*, 27(2), 203–211.

Patni, R. 2007. Communication in Practice, edited by T. Okitikpi & C. Aymer, *The Art of Social Work Practice*. Lyme Regis: Russell House Publishing, 71–85.

Reason, P. 1994. *Participation in Human Inquiry*. London: Sage.

Chapter 11

Everyday Sexuality and Identity: De-differentiating the Sexual Self in Social Work

Priscilla Dunk-West

Introduction

Social workers regularly explore service users' personal information including their backgrounds and upbringing, their attitudes and values, as well as the nature of their familial and intimate relationships. The social work assessment is broadly conceived of as providing the necessary signposts or categories for capturing important information about differing aspects of one's life. Compartmentalizing identity in this way helps social workers identify areas for concern and action. Indeed, assessments tend to highlight areas of pathology, and if details about one's intimate relationships are covered in the assessment, it is likely to be because it is an area for concern. Social workers do not routinely ask people to explain their sexual or intimate relationships or identities. Yet, in our contemporary world, in which sexual mores have evolved away from their traditional ties with reproduction, sexuality is increasingly being seen as important in social work. How those in helping professions ought to deal with the details about their clients' intimate lives has been of interest in contemporary scholarship in social work (for example, see Bywater & Jones 2007, Hafford-Letchfield 2008, Trotter & Leech 2003). Intrinsic to considerations of the sexual self and one's identity, however, has been the assumption that people may cogently speak about their sexuality without connectedness to a broader personal biography. If we argue that clients' intimate relationships and sexual selves are important to explore in contemporary assessment processes, it is important to know whether the assessment process itself is suited to the way identity is thought about in our late modern times. This involves asking whether we can separate out our sexuality from a broader identity.

This chapter reports on my recent empirical work in which thirty participants were asked to talk about their sexual selves. Through analysis of research data it was found that participants saw their biographies and wider identities as enmeshed with their sexual selves. The reflexive processes which participants engaged in to both create and sustain differing aspects of their selves draws from what I have termed as a 'de-differentiated self'. The de-differentiated self involves seeing sexuality only as part of one's biography and identity. I theorize that participants can be seen to have responded to the complexities inherent in late modern life by traversing across traditionally erected identity categories. This way of seeing identity has importance to social work theorizing as well as practice, and some of the key implications for social work are considered in this chapter. Specifically this entails exploring assessment as the means through which identity is captured. Assessment, as a method and process central to social work, is therefore examined in light of the new appreciation of self-identity.

We begin this chapter by exploring in a little more detail the late-modern notion of reflexivity as it relates to identity generally. The research design, methods and findings as well as the theoretical underpinnings of the study are then outlined. I move on to examine how the study impacts upon current understandings of the sexual self in social work. The broader implications of the de-differentiated self are explored and we consider the existing template and core social work tool: assessment. The chapter concludes by summarizing the limitations of contemporary assessment practices and approaches as well as offering some suggestions for future research and scholarship in this important area of self-identity.

Reflexivity and late modernity

I am proposing that sexuality cannot be seen as separate from other aspects of the self. Further, I suggest that should we not try to understand contemporary identity, let alone our sexual selves, without reference to key shifts in social and interpersonal life in recent times. It is such references to changes and developments in our broader social sphere that assessment processes can underplay. In considering sexuality in social work, we therefore must ask: what are the features of contemporary social life and how do these manifest in interpersonal and social life?

We live in an environment that is under constant flux: changes brought about by technological advances, shifts in communicative patterns, as well as broader developments such as globalization are all argued to have impacted upon the way we live our day-to-day lives (Beck 1992, Beck & Beck-Gernsheim 2002, Giddens 1991, Lash 2001, Urry 2003). For some, this has meant that intimate relationships are more temporary and fleeting and that without the traditional ties that once bound us to notions of duty within marriages, we have lost an important dimension to private life (Bauman 2004). For others, the flux in partnering patterns brought about by our late modern life, though both reflective and constitutive of the social milieu, has not meant the death of commitment, nor love: the ways these are manifest have simply 'transformed' (Giddens 1992). The particular forms these transformations are theorized to have taken depend on individual needs and personal requirements. Thus, relationships are negotiated based upon individuals' perceptions of self-satisfaction within the relationship (Giddens 1992). Asking oneself questions such as 'Am I happy?' 'Am I getting something from this relationship?' are examples of the thought processes involved in assessing the worth of one's relationship. In order to know whether one is happy or satisfied, however, the person must be able to engage in reflexive processes. We now move on to consider this notion of reflexivity and how this is relevant to considerations of identity and the sexual self.

As I have noted, in developed countries the ever-changing self has been argued to have been one of the central characteristics of contemporary life, and integral to the re-making of selfhood is this concept of reflexivity. The notion of reflexivity is not new to social work. It can be seen in literature, for example, that relates the dynamic and fluid learning processes that students engage in when synthesizing theory and practice (Bogo & Vayda 1987). Yet reflexivity needs to be considered in a wider context to be broadly understood in relation to identity.

Reflexivity is a signifier for the nature of our constantly changing life, which can be seen to be manifest in both internalized and external, or social, processes. As Giddens notes: '[t]he reflexive project of the self ... consists in the sustaining of coherent, yet continuously revised, biographical narratives' (1991:5). Yet how do individuals engage in these processes?

One need only turn to popular culture to witness the ubiquity of revising one's biographical narratives. Celebrity culture, for example, in advertising has meant that aspirations for self-change are targeted through products that are positioned as pivotal to transformation (Kamins 1990). The global phenomenon of the popular reality television programme, Big Brother, documents individuals engaging in reflexive deliberations and sharing these processes with others. Viewers are given a snapshot of participants' identities at the beginning of the show and invited to witness the fleshing out and transformation of individuals as they explore and test out their identities and self-hood within the confines of the 'house'. Relating narratives of themselves to the strangers with whom they are sharing space is encouraged through the deployment of games, competitions and, arguably, alcohol and 'house rules'. Having no television to watch or books to read or paper to write with also promotes a physical environment conducive to conversation and self-disclosure. Television viewers watch as contestants explore their identities over the number of months in which the show is delivered, only to emerge back into a social sphere where they can reflexively deliberate about their Big Brother experience live on national television.

There are many complexities relating to identity exploration in the media and public spheres. For example, the question of the ethics of blending private and public space and compromising individual freedoms are challenged by the Big Brother format: so much so in Greece and Belgium that '[...] regulatory agencies intervened and made recommendations to the producers and broadcasters in the name of the protection of human dignity' (Frau-Meigs 2006:48). However what Big Brother and shows of a similar kind show us is how identity is formed and re-formed. The conversations in which participants reflect upon themselves, experiment with different identities and speak about self-change and transformation, illustrate not only reflexive processes but also are evocative of the social and global contexts in which these occur. Yet how do ordinary individuals (that is, those not on television) make sense of their identities and in particular, their sexual selves?

Researching everyday sexuality: design, methods and findings

The sexuality that is experienced in day-to-day life is what I have referred to elsewhere as individual, 'everyday sexuality' (Dunk 2007). The everyday level of analysis signifies a shift to the 'ordinariness' of social phenomena and recent scholarship has seen a turn towards the everyday (Gardiner 2008). Thus,

> [...] what has come to be known as 'everyday life studies' concerns itself with the supposition that to focus exclusively on the memorable, highly visible or extraordinary events of the sociocultural world is something akin to a category mistake, because to do so universalizes the atypical and ignores the overlooked norm (Gardiner 2004:229).

Everyday sexuality involves seeing people's intimate lives as unique yet mundane and this is a counterpoint to approaches in which sexuality is attributable to difference or pathology. In social work, the everyday dimension to experience has been neglected due to an orientation towards 'difficult' sexuality (Dunk 2007), whether this be deviant sexuality (see Heap 2003) or risky sexuality (Mort 1986, Ryan 2005).

Recent empirical work in both gender and sexuality reflect an interest in the everyday (for example, see Chisholm 2008, Morrissey & Higgs 2006, Tyler 2004, Wilton 2004), though to date there have been no studies in which individual, everyday sexuality is considered using identity theories to frame the findings. There is a clear need for empirical work in this area because identity theories allow for us to think about not only our everyday lives but our lives in relation to our broader social setting. As Jackson notes, investigating the everyday allows us to make connections and see patterns. She says:

> We need ... to understand more about the ordinary day-to-day patterns of sexual relations through/in which most people life their lives (Jackson 2008:34).

Since we know so little about how and what ordinary people think and feel about their sexualities (Jackson 2008), empirical work in the area of day-to-day sexuality provides an opportunity to better understand contemporary identity in relation to one's sexual self.

As the eminent sociologist Anthony Giddens (1992) argues, in late modern life sexuality has taken on new significance for individuals. With the complex interplay of various economic and broader social changes, subjective life is theorized to be characterized by an increased awareness of self-identity. Invariably, this affects one's sexuality.

Giddens positions the sexual self as

> [...] something each of us 'has', or cultivates, [and is] no longer a natural condition which an individual accepts as a preordained state of affairs (1992:15).

Yet Giddens also points out that day-to-day individual sexuality needs elucidation. Specifically, we know little about how individuals perceive life events in contemporary society and the ways in which these experiences impact upon one's sexual self. Better understanding of this is important. He says:

> Somehow, in a way that has to be investigated, sexuality functions as a malleable feature of self, a prime connecting point between body, self-identity and social norms (Giddens 1992:15).

Giddens' (Giddens 1992) 'reflexive project of the self' speaks from the perspective of day-to-day life because these everyday practices and intimate relationships are theorized (Crook 1998). Additionally, in late modern life, reflexivity is argued to be a part of the everyday (see Adams 2006, Adkins 2003). My empirical work sought to understand how individuals made sense of their sexual selves through dialogue with research participants in which reflections about their sense-making about sexuality could be heard and understood.

Unstructured interviews (Gilbert 2001) were conducted with thirty participants, which consisted of fifteen women and fifteen men. The mean age for male participants was 44.8 years and for female participants, 43.7 years. Snowballing sampling (Biernacki and Waldorf 1981) was used as a recruiting method. Studying everyday sexuality was comparable with typical case sampling because this approach seeks to avoid selecting 'atypical' or 'deviant' populations (Patton 2002: 236). Although this study was small scale and non-representative, it provided an opportunity to investigate, in great depth, how individuals think about their sexual selves. The findings allow us to rethink social work assessment in relation to the sexual self and identity.

Findings: sexuality and broader identity

In order to explain their sexualities or sexual selves, participants involved in this study recounted other manifestations of identity that traditionally can be seen to fall outside what we might consider to be relevant to one's sexuality. In other words, sexuality was explicable only in relation to other identities in subjective and social life: the sexual self was contingent upon other realms of experience and identity. For example, I asked Ruth if she could describe her sexual self. Ruth responded with describing items of clothing – such as boots – that held symbolic meaning for her sexuality. In particular, it is the response from others within a work setting that propels Ruth to reflect upon her sexuality as well as her broader identity. The reaction of others enables her to explore her own self in which narratives relating to her gender, her sexuality, her work persona and the broader organizational context she finds herself in are all intertwined. She says:

[…] like the boots that I've got on today. I remember, I've had these boots for about 6 years. The first time I ever wore them I remember someone saying to me 'Oh you can't wear those in this environment' 'why not?' 'well they're fuck off boots, aren't they?' you know, and I'm like 'no, they're my boots and I like them and I'm going to wear them'. You know, there is no flesh showing, but yes, they are leather boots that come all the way up to my knees. And I like them![…]Um, you know, I'm a heterosexual person, um, and having been questioned by partners in the past on um, 'cause I'm quite a conservative dresser- I don't tend to be any way outlandish in my dress, um but often because depending on – especially shorter term relationships in that sort of period of time (because they were never going to last) that notion of, um, when you spend the majority of your days, I don't know different now that I'm in this sort of environment but I did work in the private sector and I've worked in the education sector and I've worked in the federal government where very very significantly male dominated so everything I did would be surrounded by, you know, well-suited, well-heeled, successful well-off blokes, which is quite threatening and can sometimes then have an impact on me and how you balance all of that out and how you see yourself in those different roles. (Ruth, 39 years, Executive Director)

It is only through looking at Ruth's entire response that one gains a sense of the connection between dressing, work and her sexual self. In fact it was only through another, important identity of 'worker' that Ruth *was able* to convey the complexities and tensions inherent in her sexual self. Removed from the private sphere most often associated with intimacy, Ruth's depiction of how clothing, gender and power played out within the work context all provided important threads in which the narrative of sexuality could come together.

For other participants, the cultural dimension to the workplace impacted upon their sexual selves in that it was the professional sphere that, to some extent, dictated how relationships were forged. Emile, for example, recounts the demographic and sheer number of the workers as being significant to the work culture.

And back to that school idea where it is kind of a social phenomenon, being overtly sexual, in my twenties I worked at the Casino which is where I met my wife and it was just like going back to school. Because you had, I think there was three or four hundred employees all of similar ages, a lot of them were single and it was just like being back at school. It was just ridiculous. (Emile, 32 years, Primary Carer for son)

For Rowan, he and his fellow workers engaged in sexual experimentation within the workplace. Employed at the time as a sessional worker in a ski resort, Rowan describes how the geographical space and social norms of the work environment lent itself to exploratory sexual behaviour.

[…] a ski bum […] The sexuality aspect of that, I was suddenly in a very sexualized environment. There was a lot of drugs. There was a lot of alcohol. And there was a lot of sex. And the first girl I hooked up with there was bisexual which led to threesomes and just this very anything goes kind of situations you have. And things that you became more, that originally I would have thought would take a while to get to this point were now very common. You know, um groups of people were having sex in the same room. We were going out and we knew that part of the room was going to be a bunch of people were going to having sex in the spa and we were going to be watching each other and you know that was part of the thing. I really I was actually I was very comfortable with my sexuality at that point. […] Very much my definition of myself at [resort name] was being that kind of guy. (Rowan, 34 years, Youth Worker)

We have seen in the above accounts the diverse ways that the workplace and the sexual self were experienced. In each of the excerpts, we can see the way that participants mapped out the relationship between their identities as workers and their sexual identities. The centre-stage position that work plays in everyday life may have meant that drawing connections between sexuality and work is not significant enough to warrant a reconfiguration of the way we think about sexuality were it not for the fact that other identities were similarly drawn upon by participants. These included differing roles played through participation in sport, religion and spiritual activities as well as experiences with formal and informal educative structures seemingly unrelated to the sexual self. For Davina, Marijka and Jane for example, theories encountered through university studies meant that they were able to reflect upon and transform their sexual and gendered selves. They explain specifically how this occurred in the following accounts that describe the synergistic coming together of ideological and theoretical ideas with personal experience and self identity. The result for each of these women was a 'transformed' identity. For Davina, this transformation came at a time when she was re-thinking her sexual relationships with men.

Like I think that a big part of wanting a non-monogamous relationship in my 20s was one, being at uni, um one, I had a child and was at uni, I was doing a philosophy degree and I ended up studying a lot of feminist theory and realising that I actually wasn't happy with the… way that I was understanding my sexuality and the way that I was interacting with men around my sexuality … (Davina, 39 years, Counsellor/Social Worker)

Marijka embodied the theoretical and ideological ideas: the broad scholarship of feminism translated into a personal statement and affinity which affected her very identity and sense of self. She says:

[…] finally finding feminism and saying, having the guts to say, so what I did was cut my hair I, like really extreme I think, just to make a point. I cut my hair,

> I think my partner at the time cut my hair and I had a tail and it was like oh my God, do you have to, because at the time I had curly locks, I had curly locks and, you know, beautiful clothes [....] And then grew my hair, my legs, didn't shave any more. And so, all those outward signs because I could see now, it doesn't really matter; I can do what I like. (Marijka, 53 years, Programme Manager)

Jane explains that the coming together of broader social shifts was very much a part of her making sense of her sexual identity as well as a larger sense of who she is. Religion, studies in criminology and discriminatory legislation in which same-sex sexual behaviour was prohibited all came together within the university setting. Jane explains:

> So like a very formative experience for me was university study around criminology [...] we had a choice of topic at one point and I chose to look at the laws against homosexuality. So this was in 1971 when I was only 18 or so and at ah and you know I had a background of um Catholicism and ah social justice era of Vatican 2 and era of the second wave of feminism. You know? Some very contradictory forces. But very intense ones. And so I think I was a sitting duck to really want to absorb this different way of thinking about sexuality ... (Jane, 53 years, Counsellor)

Similarly, David's sexuality would not make sense without reference to other areas of identity and ideology. Tracing the influencing factors not only to his university education, but when he undertook his education, David explains how these differing aspects of social and personal life have come together:

> [...] perceptions and self sense of my sexuality and things, I suppose the main issues there were the things that derived more from, I suppose, intellectual and / or ideological issues about issues such as monogamy and the basis for relationships and all those sorts of things. And that's, I suppose, coming from having been, having gone to uni in the late '70's into the early '80's initially just, I suppose a developing sense based upon broadly socialist themes type philosophies about the way in which people and social systems work. (David, 50 years, Social Planner)

Despite differing roles such as student and worker coming together in these accounts, identity was not depicted as simply unified. Rather, differing aspects of identity were talked about as co-existing alongside shifts and changes within people's social, political and spatial environments, and all of these areas were in dynamic interchange with one another. As one respondent, Bernadette, noted, the unification of seemingly disparate identities connects aspects from one role to other roles:

> But you know you have different faces for different occasion ... Because I don't feel that the person that I am at work is that much different from the person that

I am with my friends or the person that I am with my husband who's my lover.
(Bernadette, 34 years, Librarian)

As we have seen, participants in this study recruited other identities and roles in social life in order to explain and make sense of their sexual selves. In participants' accounts, we can see the dynamic interchange between differing spheres of experience and how external influences such as work and education prompted people to re-think their identities. These reflexive mechanisms explain the process that participants use to form their identities. Yet reflexivity alone does not account for explaining why differing identities were used to explain the sexual self. I propose that a de-differentiated identity, that is, one that sees sexuality as connected to other narratives of the self, is more in line with how individuals in the late modern age experience identity. Put simply, the de-differentiated self means seeing the various notions of identity labels such as 'mother', 'worker', 'lover', 'friend', 'student' as interconnected with one another. This is opposed to seeing the sexual self as completely distinct and cut off from other identities.

Yet what is de-differentiation? Broadly speaking, de-differentiation refers to the collapsing of previously established categories. For example, blurring the boundaries between the economy and culture (du Gay 1993) is an example of de-differentiation, and a signal for our late modern times. Paul du Gay explains that:

> [i]n contemporary British retailing there is no longer any room for the base/superstructure dichotomy. As the 'economic' folds seamlessly into the 'cultural', distinctions between 'production', 'consumption' and 'everyday life' become less clear cut (du Gay 1993:583).

Participants in my study used their roles such as worker, parent, student or lover to help explain their sexual selves. They did not distinguish, or *differentiate*, between 'selves'. Instead, they presented a de-differentiated identity. Yet why did they do this? I propose that the de-differentiated self is representative, and constitutive of, contemporary social life. Put simply: the de-differentiated self is a sign for our times. As Rojek (1993) points out, a de-differentiated social sphere is indicative of where we are historically. This is because de-differentiation

> [...] may be formally defined as the condition in which former social, economic, political, and cultural differentiations cease to obtain. It is therefore associated with ferment, restlessness, fresh sensations, stimulations and the ever-new (Rojek 1993:16).

In this next section of the chapter, we move to consider how the notion of a de-differentiated identity allows us to move on from more traditional notions of the self and sexuality. Specifically, the implications for the social work are considered.

The de-differentiated self and social work

In social work the fragmentation of differentiated spheres has been variously theorized, however broader social changes are largely framed alongside postmodern theories (Howe, 1994, Parton 1994). Yet, applying de-differentiation to notions of identity enables for broader social shifts to be considered. Specifically, in order to account for the complexity and contingent landscape of late modern everyday life, people make sense of their sexual selves by selectively referencing all aspects of social and interpersonal life. In this way, identity is more than just a collection of differing roles. Rather, it is a labyrinthine collection of interlocking narratives, recalled events and experiences. Asking someone to solely define their sexual selves for the purposes of completing a section in a social work assessment in this context then, appears to be a pointless exercise. In fact social work assessments invariably compartmentalize identity. Yet social work assessment, as both a skill and a tool, is firmly historically and ontologically grounded within the profession of social work.

Assessments in social work generally take an ecological approach (Adamson & Deverell 2009) which means that information about the individual as well as their social setting may be captured. Yet there are many aspects to our everyday lives: people live in complex relationships and settings with differing experiences of privilege and or disempowerment. Constructing categories in which these complexities can be explored, whilst beneficial, prevents the capturing of nuances or interfaces between such categories. This has an impact for sexuality because of its association with identity. Writing over twenty years ago, Vigilante and Mailick highlight the problems with compartmentalizing selfhood or identity. Specifically, they argue that

> [...] the assessment process has been constrained by social workers limiting clinical investigation to either intrapsychic components or environmental problems, thus inappropriately separating intrapsychic factors from social factors (Vigilante & Mailick 1988:101).

Yet assessment is ubiquitous in social work education and practice. This may be in part because assessments offer a practical way or 'framework' (Department of Health, 2000) in which identity can be clearly arranged. Sexuality is argued by some to be '...an important part of a thorough psychosocial history' (Cagle & Bolte 2009:233). Yet can sexuality be easily assigned to a category within an assessment? One of the criticisms Lord Laming recently made regarding social work assessment related to the 'tick box' (Laming 2009) nature of the activity.

Consider the narratives I have presented above from my research participants. How might these accounts fit with a traditional social work assessment? All of the information they provided about other areas of identity would have been excluded for not fitting under the heading of 'sexuality'. Indeed participant accounts of their sexual selves traversed so many identity categories and referenced various social elements (such as employment) that make it difficult to capture in a standardized format such as assessment formats.

Postmodern or critical approaches in social work have made significant scholarly contributions, whether this is through the re-configuring of personal action to collective action through human rights discourses (Ife 2001) or the disrupting of traditionally accepted epistemologies (Healy 2005, McDonald 2006, Pease & Fook 1999). In terms of assessment, postmodernist approaches emphasize the mutuality which characterizes the relationship between service user and worker (Fook 2002) and do better at accounting for agency than other approaches in which the social worker is cast as the 'expert'. Yet the very nature of the assessment task is to capture one's needs (Payne 2005: 107) based on a synthesized account of one's identity and selfhood. This being the case, using traditional forms of assessment in our late modern times is a somewhat flawed method of capturing one's identity, and therefore one's sexuality.

Yet if we accept that sexuality is an important dimension to one's identity and selfhood, then social work must account for its presence. Additionally, social workers need to see the sexual self as an important and legitimate dimension of human experience and selfhood (Dunk 2007). Yet how can existing methods of capturing identity account for the de-differentiation that we see in the above accounts? Case notes, genograms and other traditional ways of summarizing and communicating client information and selfhood are somewhat clunky fixtures in social work that do not easily accommodate a de-differentiated identity. Given the complex, changing nature of social life and identity, we need social work methods that enable these elements to be explored.

As we have seen earlier in this chapter, one of the key ways that we may characterize contemporary social life is by considering the conditions that exemplify late modern social and subjective life. The constant state of change that characterizes our social setting today has seen a shift in the ways in which individuals express and make sense of their personal lives and identities (see Beck 1992, Beck & Beck-Gernsheim 2002, Giddens 1991, Lash 2001, Urry 2003). Increased reflexivity, for example, has meant that we now think more about our identities than ever before (Giddens 1991). Rapid technological change is yet another feature of late modern life (Giddens 1991, Lash 2001). These two developments may be utilized in social work in order to develop new ways of exploring client identity and selfhood.

For example, establishing more creative and flexible methods in which service users might explore their selfhood, which includes their sexual selves, is one way forward. There has been some promising work in the area of identity and 'creative methods' by sociologist David Gauntlett (2007). His research entailed '… people … [being] asked to make things, and then reflect on them, rather than having to speak instant reports or 'reveal' themselves in verbal discussion' (Gauntlett 2007:92). Participants used Lego to construct metaphorical models of their identities and were invited to explain how the models related to their identities and then to complete a questionnaire. Here are two examples of how participants found the exercise. For one woman, building the model '... helped me discover my identity in new ways, see things from a different angle but it was not easy to explain it in words ...' whilst another liked the flexible nature of the materials '... because you can always go back to the construction and change, add or remove what doesn't fit. A lot easier than words' (Gauntlett 2007:165). Additionally, the visual nature of social networking sites such as Twitter and Facebook as well as their ubiquity tell us that these platforms appeal to people. Characterized by flexibility and self-design, these are further examples of a visual method that enables shifting, reflexive conceptions of identity: that is, identity can be made and remade.

In some areas of social work emerging technologies have been embraced, such as in the growing area of online counselling (Haberstroh, Duffey, Evans, Gee & Trepal 2007) as well as online support groups (Barak, Boniel-Nissim & Suler 2008). Designing pedagogy relating to sexuality for online use has also been found to be effective (Weerakoon 2003, Weerakoon & Wong 2002). There is room for further exploration into how social work might combine traditional methods with new technologies by using creative approaches that take into account the late modern social setting in which practice is immersed. It is only in understanding the current make-up of identity as well as how the sexual self is located within this that social work can hope to remain responsive to late modern life and ultimately, to the late modern de-differentiated identity I have identified.

Conclusion

This chapter has explored some of the key questions about identity and the sexual self in social work. Analysing empirical work in which participants were invited to talk about their everyday sexualities raised questions about the suitability of traditional social work methods and tools such as the social work assessment. The de-differentiated self was argued to represent late modern social life, in which identity is shifting and contingent upon structural and interpersonal experiences as well as linked to reflexive mechanisms. Whilst some suggestions for future directions in considering the sexual self, identity and social work were made, ultimately, it is only through re-coding identity in social work as de-differentiated that we may then move on to consider how best to respond to this new and shifting terrain.

References

Adams, M. 2006. Hybridizing habitus and reflexivity: towards an understanding of contemporary identity? *Sociology*, 40(3), 511–528.

Adamson, S. & Deverell, C. 2009. CAF in the country: implementing the Common Assessment Framework in a rural area. *Child & Family Social Work*, 14(4), 400–409.

Adkins, L. 2003. Reflexivity: freedom or habit of gender? *Theory, Culture & Society*, 20(6), 21–42.

Barak, A., Boniel-Nissim, M. & Suler, J. 2008. Fostering empowerment in online support groups. [doi: DOI: 10.1016/j.chb.2008.02.004]. *Computers in Human Behavior*, 24(5), 1867–1883.

Bauman, Z. 2004. *Liquid Love: On the Frailty of Human Bonds*. Cambridge: Polity Press.

Beck, U. 1992. *Risk Society*. London: Sage.

Beck, U. & Beck-Gernsheim, E. 2002. *Individualization: Institutionalized Individualism and its Social and Political Consequences*. London: Sage.

Biernacki, P. & Waldorf, D. 1981. Snowball sampling, *Sociological Methods and Research*, 10(2), 141–163.

Bogo, M. & Vayda, E. 1987. *The Practice of Field Instruction in Social Work: Theory and Process*. Toronto: Toronto University Press.

Bywater, J. & Jones, R. 2007. *Sexuality and Social Work*. Exeter: Learning Matters Ltd.

Cagle, J.G. & Bolte, S. 2009. Sexuality and life-threatening illness: implications for social work and palliative care. *Health & Social Work*, 34(3), 223–233.

Chisholm, D.D. 2008. Climbing like a girl: an exemplary adventure in feminist phenomenology. *Hypatia*, 23(1), 9–40.

Crook, S. 1998. Minotaur's and other monsters: 'everyday life' in recent social theory. *Sociology*, 32(3), 523–540.

Department of Health 2000. *Framework for the Assessment of Children in Need*.

du Gay, P. 1993. 'Numbers and souls': retailing and the de-differentiation of economy and culture. *The British Journal of Sociology*, 44(4), 563–587.

Dunk, P. 2007. Everyday sexuality and social work: locating sexuality in professional practice and education. *Social Work & Society*, 5(2), 135–142.

Fook, J. 2002. *Social Work Critical Theory and Practice*. London: Routledge.

Frau-Meigs, D. 2006. Big Brother and Reality TV in Europe: Towards a Theory of Situated Acculturation by the Media. *European Journal of Communication*. 21(33), 33–56.

Gardiner, M.E. 2004. Everyday utopianism. *Cultural Studies*, 18(2), 228–254.

Gardiner, M.E. 2008. Book Review: Andrew Light and Jonathan M Smith (eds) The Aesthetics of Everyday Life. *Cultural Sociology*, 2(3), 428–430.

Gauntlett, D. 2007. *Creative Explorations: New Approaches to Identities and Audiences*. Abingdon: Routledge.

Giddens, A. 1991. *Modernity and Self-Identity: Self and Society in the Late Modern Age*. Stanford: Stanford University Press.

Giddens, A. 1992. *The Transformation of Intimacy: Sexuality, Love and Eroticism in Modern Societies*. Stanford: Stanford University Press.

Gilbert, N. 2001. *Researching Social Life*. London: Sage.

Haberstroh, S., Duffey, T., Evans, M., Gee, R. & Trepal, H. 2007. The experience of online counseling. *Journal of Mental Health Counseling*. 29(3), 269–282.

Hafford-Letchfield, T. 2008. What's love got to do with it? Developing supportive practices for the expression of sexuality, sexual identity and the intimacy needs of older people. *Journal of Care Services Management*, 2(4), 389–405.

Heap, C. 2003. The city as a sexual laboratory: the queer heritage of the Chicago School. *Qualitative Sociology*, 26(4), 457–487.

Healy, K. 2005. *Social Work Theories in Context: Creating Frameworks for Practice*. Basingstoke: Palgrave Macmillan.

Howe, D. 1994. Modernity, postmodernity and social work. *British Journal of Social Work*, 24(5), 515–532.

Ife, J. 2001. *Human Rights and Social Work: Towards Rights-Based Practice*. Cambridge: Cambridge University Press.

Jackson, S. 2008. Ordinary sex. *Sexualities*, 11(1/2), 33–37.

Kamins, M.A. 1990. An investigation into the 'match-up' hypothesis in celebrity advertising: when beauty may be only skin deep. *Journal of Advertising*, 19(1), 4–13.

Laming, L. 2009. *The Protection of Children in England: A Progress Report*.

Lash, S. 2001. Technological forms of life. *Theory, Culture & Society*, 18(1), 105–120.

McDonald, C. 2006. *Challenging Social Work: The Context of Practice*. Basingstoke: Palgrave Macmillan.

Morrissey, G. & Higgs, J. 2006. Phenomenological research and adolescent female sexuality: discoveries and applications. *The Qualitative Report*, 11(1): 161–181.

Mort, F. 1986. *Dangerous Sexualities: Medico-Moral Politics in England Since 1830*. Routledge: London.

Parton, N. 1994. Problematics of governmnet (post) modernity and social work. *British Journal of Social Work*, 24(1), 9–32.

Patton, M. 2002. *Qualitative Research and Evaluation Methods*. California: Sage Publications.

Payne, M. 2005. *Modern Social Work Theory*. Basingstoke: Palgrave Macmillan.

Pease, B. & Fook, J. 1999. *Transforming Social Work Practice: Postmodern Critical Perspectives*. Sydney: Allen & Unwin.

Rojek, C. 1993. De-differentiation and leisure. *Society and Leisure*, 16, 15–29.

Ryan, A. 2005. From dangerous sexualities to risky sex: regulating sexuality in the name of public health, in *Perspectives in Human Sexuality*, edited by G. Hawkes & J.G. Scott. South Melbourne: Oxford University Press. 203–216.

Trotter, J. & Leech, N. 2003. Linking research, theory and practice in personal and professional development: gender and sexuality issues in social work education. *Social Work Education*, 33(2), 203–214.

Tyler, M. 2004. Managing between the sheets: lifestyle magazines and the management of sexuality in everyday life. *Sexualities*, 7(1), 81–106.

Urry, J. 2003. *Global Complexity*. Cambridge: Polity Press.

Vigilante, F.W. & Mailick, M.D. 1988. Needs-resource evaluation in the assessment process. *Social Work*, 33(2), 101–104.

Weerakoon, P. 2003. E-learning in sexuality education. *Medical Teacher*, 25(1), 13–17.

Weerakoon, P. & Wong, M. 2002. *Maximising opportunities for learning: sexuality education online.* Paper presented at the Annual International HERDSA Conference: Research and Development in Higher Education, Perth.

Wilton, T. 2004. *Sexual (Dis)Orientation: Gender, Sex, Desire and Self-Fashioning.* Basingstoke: Palgrave Macmillan.

Index

adoption 72, 141–148, 156–159
    legislation 107, 142, 156
    see also fostering and adoption
agency 63, 187
assessment 154–156, 177, 186–188

Bauman, Z. 2, 178
Beck-Gernsheim, E. 2, 84, 178, 187
Butler, J. 4, 20, 125, 158

children
    see family; fostering and adoption;
        social work, child protection
counselling 61
    online counselling 188
culture 6, 8, 20, 39, 75, 149, 163–166,
        170–172, 175
    see also race

de-differentiation 177–188
disability 11, 46, 123, 129, 147
discrimination 3, 11, 23–24, 34, 78–80,
        157, 159, 164–166

embodiment 171
emotions 124–125, 166–169, 167–169
equality monitoring 16, 22
ethics 33, 121, 123, 129–130, 179
everyday sexuality 177–188

family 1, 3, 6–7, 11, 13, 20, 22, 35, 37,
        71–72, 74–76, 78–79, 80, 81–84,
        107–108, 110–111, 113–114, 116,
        123, 126–127, 130, 132, 143, 146,
        148, 150, 157–159, 166
Featherstone, B.M. 84, 130
feminism 12–14, 24–25, 183–184
    feminist social work 13
    lesbian 14, 34
    second wave 14
    see also gender
Fish, J. 39, 47, 71, 75, 106–107, 124, 142, 166

Fook, J. 187
fostering and adoption 106–119, 141–159
Foucault, M. 4, 24
Freud, Sigmund 3

gay men 2, 5–7, 11, 14, 16–17, 22, 32–38,
        46, 71–76, 77–80, 82–85, 105–111,
        113–118, 124–125, 127–128,
        141–143, 145–148, 150, 155–159,
        164–166, 173–174
gay women 32
    see also lesbian; sexual identity,
        LGBTIQ
gender 4–5, 7–8, 11–12, 13–18, 20–25, 35,
        71–72, 83, 87, 89, 95–98, 100–101,
        106, 110, 113, 116, 118, 121–124,
        127–132, 144–146, 165, 180–183
    and caring 19, 21, 22
    and ethnicity 164
    and gender performativity 20
        see also Butler, J.
    and lesbians 14
    and management 17–18, 25
    and organisations 12–25, 89
    and pay 22
    definition 13
Giddens, A. 2–3, 20, 84, 178–179, 181,
        187, 180
globalization 12, 178
Goffman, E. 33, 36, 80
GUM (genitourinary medicine) 3, 61

heteronormativity 165–166, 175
heterosexuality 2–3, 7, 11, 15–16, 22–23,
        32–34, 46, 64–65, 71–72, 76, 78–79,
        83, 108, 110–118, 121–124, 126–
        129, 131–133, 142–143, 145–146,
        152, 155–157, 165–166, 174, 182
    see also sexual identity
Hicks, S. 3, 16, 72, 75, 106–108, 111,
        123, 113, 115, 124, 127, 141–143,
        145–147, 156, 158, 165

historical perspectives 7, 11–12, 24, 98
identity 24, 39, 74, 127–128, 166, 170,
        178–188
    spoiled identity 34–36
    see also sexual identity
intersex 2
    see also sexual identity; sexuality

Kerr/Haslam Inquiry 89–102
Kinsey, A. 4

language 52
leadership 19
lesbian 2–3, 5–7, 11, 14, 16–17, 22, 32–36,
        38, 46, 64, 71–79, 80, 82–84,
        105–118, 124–125, 127–128, 131,
        137, 141–151, 153, 155–159,
        164–166, 173–174
    and psychiatry 32
    parenting 72, 107–108
    see also gender, and caring; sexual
        identity, LGBTIQ

Masters, W.H. & Johnson V.E. 4
men *see* gender; gay men
mental health 89–91
    and LGB 33
    service users 39
    see also psychiatry

older age 4, 45–56
organisational theory 15, 36, 166–167

parenting 76–78
personalisation 38
pleasure 61–69
Plummer, K. 71, 73, 124
prejudice *see* discrimination
psychiatry 32–34, 89
    policy 39, 95
psychoanalytic perspective 3–4, 15, 33

queer 2–4

race 16, 22, 114, 147, 164–166
reflexivity 1, 12, 73, 169, 173, 178–179,
        185, 187
    and late modernity 178–179

relationships 3, 6–7, 13, 15–16, 22, 35–36,
        46, 53, 61–62, 64–66, 68, 71,
        73, 76, 84, 96, 99, 111–112, 121,
        122–129, 131–133, 143, 148, 155,
        168, 177–178, 181–182, 184,
        186–187
    marriage 84, 178
    partnerships 156
religion 8, 35–36, 170–172
researchers 20, 47, 50, 55–56, 96, 180
Rich, A. 34
risk 1, 4, 17, 20, 23, 32, 34, 36, 39, 53, 64,
        100, 125, 180

Seidman, S. 2
self *see* identity
self harm 31–40
sex *see* gender
sexology 4
sexual abuse 90–92, 93–94, 130
    whistleblowing 94
sexual harassment 12, 23–24
sexual identity
    definition 1, 52, 62
    categories 1, 163–164
    Homophobia *see* discrimination
    legislation 11, 84, 107
    LGBTIQ 15–17, 22–23, 71–85,
        105–119, 141–141–143
    see also sexuality; lesbian; gay men;
        transgender; intersex; queer;
        heterosexuality
sexual health 61–69
sexual and relationships education 65–66
sexual pleasure 6, 61–69
sexuality 1–7, 11–19, 20–22, 24–25,
        45–56, 61–62, 65–68, 74, 76, 78,
        80–84, 97, 100, 106, 110–111,
        114–115, 118, 121, 123–127,
        129–133, 142, 145–148, 156–159,
        165–166, 168–170, 174–175,
        177–188
    definition 1, 62
    see also sexual identity
sexually transmissible infections 63
social care *see* social work
social constructionism 4, 52
social policy *see* social work

social theory and gender and sexuality 20
social work 1, 55–56, 99–102,
      123–124, 131–133, 143,
      147–148, 149–159
   assessment 24–25, 41, 55–56, 84,
      105–107, 109–118, 127–128,
      142–143, 147–149, 151–159,
      177–188
   child protection 116, 125–126, 130, 142
   codes of practice 129–130, 132
   education 163–175
   postmodern social work 187
   social care 11, 14, 16–19, 21–25,
      39–40, 51, 83, 96, 100–101, 106,
      124–125, 129
   social policy 12, 18–19, 39–40, 45, 56,
      71, 84, 90, 94–95, 98, 100–102,
      107, 121, 127, 133

Stonewall 16, 35
substance misuse 32

therapeutic culture 3–4, 37
transgender 2, 7, 22, 106, 124, 166
   see also sexual identity, LGBTIQ

violence 15, 24, 35, 78, 95, 97, 100, 126,
   132
   domestic violence 13, 66, 130
   see also discrimination

Wakefield enquiry 108–110, 117
Weeks, J. 71, 73, 108, 113
women *see* gender

young people 63, 75–82
young women 66–67, 74